W9-BTT-538

The Role of Epidemiology
in Regulatory Risk Assessment

The Role of Epidemiology in Regulatory Risk Assessment

Proceedings of the Conference on the Proper Role of Epidemiology in Risk Analysis, Boston, MA, U.S.A., 13–14 October 1994

Edited by:

John D. Graham
Director, Center for Risk Analysis
Harvard School of Public Health
Boston, Massachusetts, USA

 1995

ELSEVIER

Amsterdam – Lausanne – New York – Oxford – Shannon – Tokyo

©1995 Elsevier Science B.V. All rights reserved.

No part of this publication may be reproduced, stored in a retrieval system or transmitted in any form or by any means, electronic, mechanical, photocopying, recording or otherwise without the prior written permission of the publisher, Elsevier Science B.V., Permissions Department, P.O. Box 521, 1000 AM Amsterdam, The Netherlands.

No responsibility is assumed by the Publisher for any injury and/or damage to persons or property as a matter of products liability, negligence or otherwise, or from use or operation of any methods, products, instructions or ideas contained in the material herein. Because of rapid advances in the medical sciences, the Publisher recommends that independent verification of diagnoses and drug dosages should be made.

Special regulations for readers in the USA — This publication has been registered with the Copyright Clearance Center Inc. (CCC), 222 Rosewood Drive, Danvers, MA 01293, USA. Information can be obtained from the CCC about conditions under which photocopies of parts of this publication may be made in the USA. All other copyright questions, including photocopying outside the USA should be referred to the copyright owner, Elsevier Science B.V., unless otherwise specified.

ISBN 0 444 82201 1

This book is printed on acid-free paper.

Published by:
Elsevier Science B.V.
P.O. Box 211
1000 AE Amsterdam
The Netherlands

Library of Congress Cataloging-in-Publication Data:

In order to ensure rapid publication this volume was prepared using a method of electronic text processing known as Optical Character Recognition (OCR). Scientific accuracy and consistency of style were handled by the author. Time did not allow for the usual extensive editing process of the Publisher.

Printed in the Netherlands

List of contributors

Thorne Auchter
Director
Institute for Regulatory Policy
11 DuPont Circle, N.W. #700
Washington, DC 20036, USA
Tel.: +1-202-939-6976
Fax: +1-202-939-6969

Gregory Bond
Health and Environmental Sciences
Dow Chemical Company
1803 Building
Midland, MI 48674, USA
Tel.: +1-517-636-9063
Fax: +1-517-636-1875

Thomas Burke
Assistant Professor of Health Policy and Management
551 Hampton House
Johns Hopkins School of Medicine
720 Rutland Avenue
Baltimore, MD 21205, USA
Tel.: +1-410-955-1604
Fax: +1-410-614-2797

William J. Butler
McLaren/Hart Chemical Risk Division
1135 Atlantic Avenue
Alameda, CA 94501, USA
Tel.: +1-510-521-5200
Fax: +1-510-521-1547

Alvan R. Feinstein
Clinical Epidemiology Unit
333 Cedar Street
Yale University School of Medicine
New Haven, CT 06510, USA
Tel.: +1-203-785-5177
Fax: +1-203-785-4146

Earl Ford
Radiation Studies Branch
National Center for Environmental Health
Centers for Disease Control and Prevention
4770 Buford Highway, NE
Mailstop F35
Atlanta, GA 30341, USA
Tel.: +1-404-488-7040
Fax: +1-404-488-7044

Christine M. Friedenreich
Department of Community Health Sciences
The University of Calgary
3330 Hospital Drive, NW
Calgary, Alberta
Canada T2N 4N1
Tel.: +1-403-220-8242 (5110)
Fax: +1-403-283-4740

Gay Goodman
California EPA
Department of Pesticide Regulation
Medical Toxicology Branch
1020 N Street
Sacramento, CA 95814, USA
Tel.: +1-916-324-3512
Fax: +1-916-324-3506

John D. Graham
Director
Harvard Center for Risk Analysis
718 Huntington Avenue
Boston, MA 02115, USA
Tel.: +1-617-432-4343
Fax: +1-617-432-0190

Linda Koo
Cancer Research Laboratory
7th Floor, Nam Long Hospital
30 Nam Long Shan Road
Wong Chuk Hang
Hong Kong
Tel.: +852-552-7923
Fax: +852-817-6528

Malcolm Maclure
Associate Professor of Epidemiology
Kresge 902
Harvard School of Public Health
677 Huntington Avenue
Boston, MA 02115, USA
Tel.: +1-617-432-1199
Fax: +1-617-566-7805

Malcolm Maclure
Research and Evaluation Branch
Ministry of Health
1515 Blanchard Street
Victoria, British Columbia
Canada V8W 3C8
Tel.: +1-604-952-2300
Fax: +1-604-952-2308

Genevieve M. Matanoski
Professor of Epidemiology
School of Hygiene and Public Health
The Johns Hopkins University
624 North Broadway, Room 280
Baltimore, MD 21205, USA
Tel.: +1-410-955-8183
Fax: +1-410-276-0290

Suresh Moolgavkar, M.D., Ph.D.
Program in Biostatistics
Fred Hutchinson Cancer Research Center
1124 Columbia Street, MP-665
Seattle, WA 98104, USA
Tel.: +1-206-667-4273
Fax: +1-206-667-7004

Dennis Paustenbach
Vice President and Chief Technical officer
McLaren/Hart Chemical Risk Division
1135 Atlantic Avenue
Alameda, CA 94501, USA
Tel.: +1-510-521-5200
Fax: +1-510-521-1547

Göran Pershagen
Department of Epidemiology
Institute of Environmental Medicine
Karolinska Institute
Box 210, S-17177 Stockholm, Sweden
Tel.: +46-468-728-6400
Fax: +46-468-313961

Lorens Rhomberg
Harvard Center for Risk Analysis
718 Huntington Avenue
Boston, MA 02115, USA
Tel.: +1-617-432-0095
Fax: +1-617-432-0190

Robert Sielken
Sielken, Inc.
3833 Texas Avenue, Suite 230
Bryan, TX 77802, USA
Tel.: +1-409-846-5175
Fax: +1-409-846-2671

Allan H. Smith
Department of Biomedical and
Environmental Health Sciences
University of California-B
Berkeley, CA 94720, USA
Tel.: +1-510-843-1763
Fax: +1-510-843-5539

Ernst L. Wynder
American Health Foundation
320 East 43rd St.
New York, NY 10017, USA
Tel.: +1-212-953-1900
Fax: +1-914-592-6317

Contents

©1995 Elsevier Science B.V. All rights reserved.
The Role of Epidemiology in Regulatory Risk Assessment
J.D. Graham, editor.

1

Epidemiology and risk assessment: divorce or marriage?*

John D. Graham[1], Dennis J. Paustenbach[2] and William J. Butler[2]
Harvard Center for Risk Analysis, 718 Huntington Avenue, Boston, MA 02115; and [2]McLaren/Hart Chemical Risk Division, 1135 Atlantic Avenue, Alameda, CA 94501, USA

Key words: assessment, epidemiology, exposure, guidelines, health, regulation, risk.

Introduction

The analytic tools of risk assessment, as applied to chemicals and radiation, have assumed a critical role in decision making in the United States. While risk assessment might appear to be an arcane subject, each day the public health, environmental resources, and the economic wellbeing of families are affected by the outcomes of risk assessment. Many jobs, new products and industrial facilities are threatened, protected or created by the outcomes of risk assessments performed by government agencies.

At the U.S. Environmental Protection Agency, for example, risk assessments play a significant role in determining how much human exposure is permitted to new chemicals, existing chemicals, pesticides, radon, hazardous wastes, toxic air pollution, drinking water contaminants and surface water pollutants. Other federal agencies that employ quantitative risk assessment include the Consumer Product Safety Commission, the Department of Defense, the Department of Energy, the Food and Drug Administration, the Nuclear Regulatory Commission, and the Occupational Safety and Health Administration. Many states, especially California, New Jersey and Wisconsin, also make widespread use of risk assessment in making public health and environmental decisions. While the U.S. approach to risk assessment is somewhat unique, many countries around the world are considering adoption of the U.S. approach or are developing their own approaches (IPCS, 1992).

In the last twenty years, principles and guidelines have been developed by the federal government that influence the conduct of risk assessment in the regulatory process. Although risk assessment guidelines vary greatly in their degree of specificity and sophistication (and some prevailing guidelines remain the subject of

---

Address for correspondence: John D. Graham, PhD, Director, Harvard Center for Risk Analysis, 718 Huntington Avenue, Boston, MA 02115, USA. Tel. +1-617-432-4343. Fax: +1-617-432-0910.
*The views presented are those of the author and not necessarily those of the Environmental Protection Agency.

heated controversy), a practicing risk assessor whether employed in the public or private sector, can frequently find useful direction in guidelines and guidance documents when preparing a formal risk assessment report.

Many types of technical information are addressed in guidelines ranging from the proper interpretation of tumor data in laboratory animal bioassays to the proper use of exposure data collected near industrial facilities that pollute air or water. Interestingly, relatively little specific direction has been provided about how epidemiological information should be utilized in quantitative risk assessment.

For example, even a cursory examination of the U.S. Environmental Protection Agency's guidelines for cancer and noncancer risk assessment will reveal far more discussion of experimental information than epidemiological information.

Although some fairly specific guidance can be found about the role of human data in the qualitative process of hazard identification (e.g., see how OSHA's generic carcinogen identification rule treats epidemiological data in relation to animal data in defining "occupational carcinogens"). But relatively little guidance addresses how numerical estimates of risk to exposed populations should be derived from a body of epidemiological information (or a mix of laboratory and epidemiological data). Similarly, the level of specificity provided in guidance documents on exposure assessment (e.g., the protocols for risk assessors to follow when predicting human exposure to contaminants at a Superfund site) are much more developed than is the available guidance about how to use epidemiological information in determining a "cancer potency factor" or "acceptable daily intake" value.

This Chapter explores whether there are sound reasons for the absence of specific guidelines about the proper use of epidemiology in regulatory risk assessment. Please let us emphasize the distinction between principles governing the proper conduct of epidemiological studies (where some specific principles have been suggested by various governmental and nongovernmental bodies) and principles governing how data derived from human studies — however well conducted — should be incorporated into quantitative estimates of risk.

Working definitions and context

By "epidemiology" we refer to the distribution and determinants of health related states or events in specified populations, and the application of (the results of) this study to control health problems (Last, 1988). It is these methods, rather than the controlled experiments that characterize laboratory science, that were successful in identifying some of the major cancer-causing effects of smoking and human exposure to ionizing radiation. More recently, these methods have drawn public attention to the potential dangers of radon in homes, chlorination of drinking water, environmental tobacco smoke, pesticide use among farmers, electric and magnetic fields near power lines, birth defects in families living near hazardous waste sites, cognitive impairment among children exposed to lead, and a variety of health impairments among workers.

This definition includes the application of epidemiologic research to control disease, which would encompass the practice of quantitative risk assessment when used to prevent disease. This definition also includes in epidemiology the study of the patterns and intensities of exposures (that is, "determinants"). Exposure assessment is an area in which epidemiology can make a substantial contribution to risk assessment either through the examination of exposure — disease relationships in humans (i.e., asbestos and lung cancer) or in providing population exposure-related information to be linked with other risk assessment data (i.e., soil consumption patterns in children). Currently, exposure assessment is one of epidemiology's weaker links. Among sixty recently published results from case-control studies of occupational and environmental agents, Correa et al. (1994) found that quantitative intensity and duration data were available from only 20 and 32% of the studies, respectively. The absence of exposure information is probably the leading reason why risk assessments are based on animal bioassay data even when epidemiologic data are available to support the conclusion of human carcinogenicity. Improvements in exposure assessment will substantially increase the utility of both epidemiologic and toxicologic research for the quantitative risk assessment.

By "risk assessment" we refer to the analytic process of combining information on the presence or extent of human exposure to environmental agents with data on health effects (whether drawn from epidemiology and/or laboratory studies) to predict the probability (or frequency) of health effects in a population. Unlike the science of epidemiology, which explores health effects that may occur from exposures within a specific region of empirical observation (e.g., a study of these health effects from these levels of exposures experienced by male workers in this age group), risk assessment usually entails prediction of the frequency of health responses outside the range of empirical observation based on the frequency observed in the study population. The exposures of interest to risk assessors may involve different contexts or subjects than were studied by epidemiologists, or they may simply involve magnitudes or patterns of exposure that are outside the epidemiologist's region of observation.

By philosophy, the epidemiologist is inclined to inquire whether a cause-effect relationship between an agent and health effects is known (or not) based on available data (Monson, 1990); the risk assessor, recognizing that decisions often must be made before the cause-effect link is revealed with certainty, is inclined to offer speculative risk estimates — usually assuming causation — that cannot be verified with available data (Rodericks, 1992). Although there is a community of experts that practice both epidemiology and risk assessment, this community is quite small (just as the overlap between toxicologists and risk assessors is limited).

A "regulatory" risk assessment is an official report (or series of reports) issued by a government agency that describes this analytic process and the results. Although risk assessment *per se* is not regulation, it is an analytic process that is often critical in the development and defense of actions taken by regulatory agencies. For example, the federal courts have ruled that OSHA may not regulate a contaminant in the work place unless a risk assessment demonstrates that the risk may be significant (Graham et al., 1988).

The publicity about the findings of a risk assessment report (even prior to or without any regulation) can also have an informal yet influential impact in society. In some cases, the mere publication of an official risk assessment report, and the associated publicity in the mass media and trade journals, can have major consequences for both public health and the fate of specific technologies or products, even if a regulatory agency decides to take no formal rule making action. For example, in 1994 the release of EPA's draft risk assessment report on dioxin received widespread television coverage and front-page billing in the print media. This publicity can have profound societal impacts. Not only can an official risk determination have important liability implications in common law (e.g., when an attorney in a tort liability suit claims that a product is dangerous or safe based on findings in an official risk assessment report), it can also have competitive implications in the marketplace as technologies compete for customer loyalty (e.g., official reports about the human health risks of chemical pest control may promote the development of biotechnology-based products and organic foods).

We now return to the question of whether guidelines are needed to inform the risk assessor's use of epidemiological data in quantitative risk assessment. The question is addressed by considering the validity of two reasons why such guidelines are not needed or appropriate. We conclude by discussing why the development of such guidelines, difficult as they may be to construct, cannot be avoided for much longer. At the same time, we acknowledge dangers in the development of guidelines that are overly descriptive or inflexible.

Myth 1. Since epidemiological information is rarely relevant to important risk assessments and the related activities of regulatory agencies, it is not worth the effort to develop specific guidelines covering epidemiology.

It is certainly true that only a small fraction of quantitative risk assessments make direct use of epidemiological information. This fact is revealed by a review of the quantitative risk information contained in U.S. EPA's Integrated Risk Information Service (IRIS). For cancer effects, the critical number in IRIS is a chemical's "slope factor" or potency factor, which is the incremental probability of contracting cancer from a standardized 70-year exposure to 1 microgram per cubic meter of the chemical. For noncancer effects, the critical number is the "reference concentration" (inhalation) or "reference dose" (oral), which represents an estimated daily exposure or intake that is sufficiently small that there are unlikely to be any adverse effects in the exposed population — sometimes called the "acceptable daily intake".

Of the 520 chemicals in the IRIS database as of June 1994, only 11 of the 218 evaluated for cancer have numerical slope factors that are based entirely or partially on epidemiological data. These chemicals are acrylonitrile, inorganic arsenic, asbestos, benzene, benzidine, beryllium, cadmium, chromium (IV), coke oven emissions, nickel refinery dust, and nickel subsulfide. In IRIS only benzene and benzidine have cancer slope factors for both oral and inhalation exposure. Acrylonitrile and beryllium have inhalation slope factors based on human data but the oral slope factors are based on animal data. The other seven chemicals have inhalation slope factors based on human data but have no reported oral slope factor.

Inhalation reference concentrations in IRIS are available for 88 chemicals, only six of which are based on human data. They are ammonia, n,n-dimethylformamide, n-hexane, manganese, styrene and toluene. Oral reference doses in IRIS are available for 348 chemicals, only 27 of which are based on human data. In some cases the reference concentrations or reference doses are based on experimental human studies (e.g., clinical trials) rather than epidemiology as defined at the outset of the paper.

Based on this survey of IRIS chemicals, one might be tempted to discount the importance of epidemiology in risk assessment and regulatory decisions. This conclusion would be too hasty.

First, epidemiology plays a crucial role in risk assessments and regulation of several ubiquitous pollutants that are not contained in IRIS. For example, federal agencies routinely use epidemiological information to assess the cancer risks of low-level exposures to ionizing radiation. These assessments now inform multibillion dollar investments in risk management at nuclear power plants, abandoned weapon sites, uranium mines, and residential homes and buildings where radon is present. The estimated risks of skin cancer from stratospheric ozone depletion, which were based on epidemiological data about the effects of exposure to ultraviolet radiation, also played an important role in the international treaties restricting the widespread use of chlorofluorocarbons and other ozone-depleting agents. Moreover, the so-called "criteria air pollutants" (lead, carbon monoxide, nitrogen dioxide, fine particles, sulphur dioxide and tropospheric ozone) are assessed and regulated by EPA through a separate health assessment process that makes substantial use of epidemiological information. EPA's regulatory program for criteria pollutants, which includes complex implementation plans in every state and stringent rules on motor vehicle engines and fuels, represents another multibillion dollar program of pollution prevention and control.

Second, there are several important complex mixtures (not contained in IRIS) that are assessed and regulated by EPA at least partly on the basis of epidemiological information. The most publicized example, EPA's recent risk assessment of environmental tobacco smoke, is now a driving force in the USA behind a surge of federal, state and local policies aimed at curbing smoking. Concern about ETS is also prodding OSHA to consider serious regulation of indoor air pollution. A less publicized assessment by California EPA, the one addressing cancer risk from exposure to diesel exhaust from motor vehicles, is based partly on epidemiological data and may play a crucial role in determining the future of diesel-powered vehicles in the United States.

Third, several of the cancer slope factors reported in IRIS that are based on human data play a major role in multibillion dollar regulatory programs. Most notable in this respect is benzene, where epidemiological evidence is the primary basis of numerous rule makings whose annual costs are in the billion-dollar range. At Superfund sites and under the Safe Drinking Water Act, the cancer slope factor and reference dose for inorganic arsenic are driving major economic investments by states and localities and private industry. The annual U.S. investment in control of benzene and arsenic exposures alone might very well be larger than the investment associated with controlling a random sample of 100 of the other IRIS chemicals.

Fourth, risk estimates derived from rodent data are far from perfect (Lave et al., 1988). Attempts to validate the qualitative and quantitative correspondence between animal and human cancer potency factors have not been completely satisfactory (Allen et al., 1988; Gold, Manley and Ames, 1992). The most recent review on a quantitative correspondence (Allen et al., 1988) is now dated, and a new evaluation of the correspondence of toxicologic and epidemiologic findings would be most welcome. Though there is, in general, a positive correlation between the list of rodent and human carcinogens, a sufficient amount of error remains to warrant substantial investments in epidemiologic research methods either to avoid the need for or to validate interspecies extrapolations. Moreover, standard animal bioassays and most toxicology, testing protocols provide limited data on important aspects of the exposure-risk relationship such as the dependency of risk on chronological age at exposure; dose dependent pharmaconetics; intermittent versus continuous exposure patterns; concomitant exposure to other agents; and variability of response in genetically heterogeneous populations. Epidemiologic studies provide the opportunity to collect data on each of these topics (Kaldor, 1992) though at times the quantitative information on these issues may be limited or need to be obtained indirectly.

Fifth, epidemiology can provide some unique information that toxicologists cannot supply. A prominent example is the assessment of the fit of the multistage model for carcinogenesis to human cancer mortality data (Armitage and Doll, 1961) which was central to its acceptance for low-dose extrapolation in animals and humans. Epidemiologic data are also likely to be important in choosing between different biologically based extrapolation models such as the multistage model or the two-stage clonal expansion model. Historically, there has been limited confidence in the estimates of risk from models since the results were often clearly inconsistent with the epidemiologic experience. Epidemiology is unique in its ability to detect rare adverse reactions to occupational exposures, pharmaceutical agents and medical devices. Examples include the association of asbestos with mesothelioma, aspirin with Reye's Syndrome in children, a mother's exposure to DES with adenocarcinoma of the vagina in her daughters and intrauterine devices with decreased fertility. For pharmaceutical agents, these types of associations are unlikely to be detected or refuted through the extensive toxicologic studies and clinical trials conducted prior to FDA approval. Epidemiologic monitoring of adverse drug reactions and occupational surveillance systems may be the only means to detect and examine these rare events that may occur only in small subsets of a susceptible population. Moreover, epidemiologic designs, unlike those in toxicology testing, can assess the risks of injuries (as opposed to disease) related to consumer and work place products. Injuries to all-terrain vehicles, baby walkers and the structure of jobs (that is, ergonomic requirements) have all received substantial national attention. Each of these topics has been studied using the same epidemiologic study designs and principles used to evaluate chemical agents though, admittedly, questions related to the validity of high-to-low dose extrapolation would not apply.

Finally, and perhaps most importantly, there are good reasons to believe that epidemiological information will play a more important role in future risk assessments than it has in the past. Growing skepticism about the relevance and ethics of standard animal testing may induce risk assessors and regulators to give more credence to even imperfect epidemiological data. Meanwhile, the development of biological markers of human exposure and effects may make it possible to perform prospective epidemiogical studies in a way that was not possible even ten years ago. A host of large-scale epidemiological studies of modern life are now in progress — studies addressing electric and magnetic fields near power lines, cellular telephones, video display terminals, pesticide exposures among farmers, and community exposures to contaminants at abandoned hazardous waste sites — that will surely produce findings that demand consideration by risk assessors. At the very least, the future of quantitative risk assessment would appear to demand some creative syntheses of information from epidemiological and experimental studies.

Myth 2. Since there is little analytical discretion and few controversies about how to use epidemiological data in risk assessment, guidelines are not necessary.

Even if epidemiology is judged to be important to risk assessment and regulation, guidelines are unnecessary if the proper use of this information by risk assessors is obvious. Based on the limited experience to date, this assumption seems very dubious.

For starters, it is far from obvious when epidemiology should be used in quantitative risk assessment if "positive" findings from both rodents and people are available. In the case of cancer risk from exposure to diesel exhaust, the U.S. EPA chose rodent data while California EPA chose epidemiological data. Formaldehyde is a case where U.S. EPA relied primarily on animal data in cancer risk assessment but was criticized by the Agency's Science Advisory Board for not making more use of occupational epidemiology data. Human cancer risk from dioxin exposure has traditionally been derived from rodent data but some would argue that the human data are becoming sufficiently informative to justify a slope factor based on epidemiology. In its butadiene risk assessment, U.S. EPA relies on rodent data but the National Institute of Occupational Safety and Health (NIOSH) has published risk assessment reports that use both animal and human data. When similar risk estimates are generated from animal and human data, there is no real dilemma but controversy arises when this fortunate circumstance does not occur.

Part of the controversy for these agents involves the proper execution and interpretation of epidemiologic studies, rather than the lack of guidelines and is not specific to the use of epidemiology for quantitative risk assessment. Examples of continued epidemiologic controversy for formaldehyde are presented by Sterling and Weinkam (1994) and Blair and Stewart (1994) and for butadiene are presented by Cole, Delzell and Acquavella (1993), Park (1993), and Matanoski and Santos-Burgoa (1994).

Instructions on epidemiologic methods and principles are provided not only in excellent textbooks and monographs but also in guidelines generated by industrial associations (Epidemiology Task Group, 1991). Further, Hill's (1965) guidelines for assessing causality have served epidemiologists in the planning and interpretation of their studies and have not been challenged or improved upon. More recently, epidemiologists have given particular emphasis to the consideration of low-risk agents (Samet, 1990; Acquavella et al., 1994) and to the interpretation of negative epidemiologic evidence for carcinogenicity (Wald and Doll, 1985; Elcock and Morgan, 1993). The much needed guidelines for the use of epidemiologic research in quantitative risk assessment should build from these existing guidance documents that are currently available to and relied upon by the epidemiologic research community.

Even if there is agreement that "positive" human data should be used, it is often far from clear how this information should be used to compute low-dose risk. If epidemiologists report only responses for those "exposed" versus those "unexposed", should risk assessors make more speculative groupings of subjects by judged degrees of exposure and fit a dose-response curve? Should risk assessors be restricted to the information reported by epidemiologists in their published papers or should they be free to ask of (or expect from) authors their complete data bases? If the dose-response curve is clearly nonlinear within the range of observation (as has been observed for coke oven emissions and some radiation effects), what dose-response shape should be used to extrapolate responses below the range of empirical observation? If more than one epidemiological study is available, should risk assessors use only the "best" or "most sensitive" study or should they pool data from multiple studies in risk estimation? If forms of "meta-analysis" are to be used, should guidance be available to risk assessors on the proper procedures to employ when excluding or weighting studies? Based on interviews with several risk assessors and epidemiologists in state and federal regulatory agencies, we learned that these kinds of questions (and many others) need to be asked because the answers to them are important but not always obvious.

The proper use of "negative" or "nonpositive" epidemiological data in quantitative risk assessment is also far from obvious. EPA's 1986 cancer risk assessment guidelines state that "if adequate exposure data exist in a well-designed and well-conducted negative epidemiologic study, it may be possible to obtain an upper-bound estimate of risk from that study." Yet we found no case in the IRIS database where a rodent-based slope factor was adjusted downward because of the insight provided by a negative epidemiological study. While this may simply reflect the weak statistical power of epidemiological studies, it may also reflect ambiguity about when a study is good enough to justify this kind of adjustment. Our colleague Bernard Goldstein has commented that this calculation of an upper bound based on negative human data, if it is routinely made, is certainly not reported routinely in official risk assessment reports.

What should be in the guidelines?

Dose Response Assessment

One essential component for guidelines on the application of epidemiology to risk assessment is the selection and estimation of the appropriate dose-response models. Typically, epidemiological data are analyzed with statistically based multiplicative models (for example, logistic regression) that are convenient for data description (Breslow et al., 1983; Becher and Wahrendoff, 1990). Such models have been extremely useful for examining multivariate patterns of disease frequency but differ from the biologically based risk assessment models used for extrapolation. Realistically, a shift to the routine use of the risk assessment models by epidemiologists is unlikely to occur until guidance is more readily available and the models are shown to provide insight into important epidemiologic features such as the confounding, age-dependency of risk, and the joint exposure to carcinogens. The absence of quantitative exposure data, mentioned earlier, is one reason for the infrequent use of the epidemiologic data to establish estimates of human risk. The credibility of the entire risk assessment process would be much improved if epidemiology were used to help validate the results for risk assessments. For example, when one examines the risks predicted by low-dose models to occupational standards and guidelines (such as PELs or TLVs), one does not have confidence that they reflect reality. It is clear that the epidemiologic data are not consistent with the risks predicted by animal studies and the linearized multistage model for agents such as TCDDs, inorganic arsenic, asbestos, and others (Leung and Paustenbach, 1988).

Retrospective Exposure Assessments

Guidelines will help accelerate on-going efforts to improve the quality and to increase the quantification of exposure assessments used in epidemiology studies (Armstrong et al., 1992; Rappaport and Smith, 1991; Paustenbach et al., 1992; Hawkins, 1992). The construction of job-exposure matrices seems to be the method of choice to examine dose-response relationships for occupational agents and might be considered as the structure on which to provide guidance on exposure assessment. Quantitative industrial hygiene information is often available for substantial portions of such a matrix, though direct information may be sparse for the exposure intensities from the more distant past. Due to latency issues, the historical exposures are of prime interest but, unfortunately, are usually estimated with the least precision and the most uncertainty. To supplement the direct measurements of the agent of interest, it is essential to consider the use of indirect information on exposure such as direct industrial hygiene measurements of similar occupational agents; personal interviews with surviving workers and managers; production, sales and shipping information; plant purchasing records; concomitant frequency of related diseases; local industrial hygiene controls such as ventilation; effectiveness of personal protection devices such as respirators; and medical evidence of overexposure (Paustenbach et al., 1992).

Guidance might be offered in the use of these types of sources to provide a basis to impute entries into cells of the job-exposure matrix for which direct measurements are not available. These guidelines might help epidemiologists to overcome their reluctance to use imperfect data for risk assessment (Whittemore, 1986; Omenn, 1993). We believe that epidemiologists are quite willing for these data to be used in such settings (Checkoway, 1993).

The uncertainty in risk assessments based on job-exposure matrices calculated with imputations can be assessed through Monte Carlo simulations and the more sensitive factors can be identified for further investigation. Different assumptions and imputations into the dose reconstruction can have a substantial impact on the slope of the estimated exposure response relationship, as well as on the calculation of cancer potency factors, from epidemiologic studies (Crurnp et al., 1994). However, this uncertainty will usually not be as great as that resulting from interspecies extrapolations based on bioassays that do not represent the exposure patterns experienced by humans (Allen et al., 1988). Further, the uncertainty in epidemiologic studies can be mathematically assessed and, if necessary, additional data on historical information can be pursued to reduce the overall uncertainty.

The guidance document should also reflect that precise exposure assessments are particularly important for agents for which human exposure may be from multiple sources and be associated with low risks. Examples include; a) the developmental abnormalities in children from exposure to lead from paint, dust, soil, water, air and food; and b) respiratory disease from exposure to benzo(a)pyrene from smoking, food, cooking sources and ambient air pollution. Since regulatory criteria are usually media-specific, it is necessary to determine the relative contribution and risk for each of the multiple sources of exposure. For example, remediation programs to remove lead paint from households of children may not be the best use of resources if tap water or exterior soil were found to be the major sources of lead.

Issues of Bias

Similarly, guidance on the needs for and methods to assess potential bias from confounding and misclassification should be included. We think this is particularly important when epidemiologic research uses imprecise measures of exposure to agents that have low magnitudes of risk. Examples include environmental tobacco smoke and electromagnetic fields. Confounding is less of a consideration when specific biomarkers of specific exposures are found to have large magnitudes of association with specific diseases.

The elimination of all confounding or other bias can never be achieved, but the *quantification* of the possible amount of confounding from reasonable sources should be undertaken when epidemiologic studies are used for risk assessment. For example, smokers have different diets and lifestyles than do nonsmokers, and these factors are associated with lung cancer mortality. However, the expected degree of confounding from these factors is not of a magnitude to explain the very large relative risks with smoking. On the other hand, the relative risk between ETS and lung cancer is much smaller and could be due (in whole or in substantial part) to the documented dietary, lifestyle and other health differences associated with the surrogate measures of ETS exposure that have been used in these studies. A similar argument can be developed for occupational and environmental studies of EMF. We agree with Hill (1965) that the emphasis in the guidelines should be on the *quantification* of the possible confounding and not just the supposition that some confounding exists. The former would be useful in a "weight of evidence" determination while the latter is nothing more than unconstructive 'epidemiology-bashing'.

Using all our resources

Population surveys by the National Centers for Health Statistics represent substantial components of the nations investment in the superstructure for epidemiology, and the full utilization of these resources should be included in quantitative risk assessments when appropriate. The decline in children's blood lead levels during the phasing out of leaded gasoline in the U.S. is a well recognized example of the contribution of these data to the evaluation of risk management choices (Annest et al., 1983). Similarly, birth defects and cancer registries represent a substantial investment in public health resources but currently provide only the crudest of information required for quantitative risk assessment (Parkin, 1985). At least one registry has attempted to link a job-exposure matrix to its case interview database, but to date only descriptive information on crude measures of exposure are available (Katz et al., 1994). Vital statistics databases can also be useful sources of information, but because only crude information is available on exposures and confounders, their analyses may be not only uninformative but distracting. Some epidemiologists have referred to analyses from these sources as "hypothesis generating machines" since the large number of statistical tests from these analysts will assuredly generate some "statistically significant" associations.

"Clusters" and Environmental Contamination

On a slightly different topic, epidemiologic studies have played a major role in the identification and investigation of disease clusters which are often suspected of being associated with environmental pollution or consumer products. A suspected cluster can be a quite disruptive event and can cause a frenzy of unproductive activities by government agencies, industrial groups, environmental activists and research scientists. Examples of such controversies include the drinking water contamination episodes in San Jose, CA (Deane et al., 1992) and in Woburn, MA (Lagakos et al., 1986). Guidelines on quantitative risk assessment for such episodes could supplement the guidelines currently available for epidemiologic investigation (Centers for Disease Control, 1990). Further, guidelines directed toward nonscientific personnel (citizen groups, labor unions, elected officials and the popular press) could contribute substantially to the prevention of unnecessary public concern and panic.

12

Conclusion

Many regulatory decisions are made and must be made without any information from epidemiology. The most obvious circumstance is regulation of new chemicals or products where the historical exposures of people have simply not occurred; in these cases experiments must be conducted to provide toxicity data for risk assessors and regulators. More generally, when epidemiology is not available or is completely uninformative, then it is sound public health practice to base regulatory decisions on risk assessments rooted in experimental toxicity information. To simply await the availability of human data would discard the preventive principles that distinguish public health from much of clinical medicine.

The central theme of this article, however, is that we have not thought hard enough about how risk assessors and regulators should use epidemiological information when it is available. The most telling indication of this syndrome is that regulatory agencies have provided practicing risk assessors with virtually no technical guidance on how to properly use epidemiological information in quantitative risk assessment.

In our view, we have no choice but to begin the intellectually challenging task of developing formal guidelines, rooted in our practical experience, to govern the use of epidemiology in risk assessment. We believe such guidelines will be welcomed by those doing epidemiologic research (Omenn, 1993; Checkoway, 1993). Segments of the public, the media, and opinion leaders are beginning to learn that, when it comes to epidemiology, risk assessment, and regulation, the emperor has no clothes.

Acknowledgements

The author acknowledges helpful comments from Stephen Baird, Chao Chen, and John Evans. Danna Felgoise provided helpful research assistance. Opinions and errors are the responsibility of the author.

References

Acquavella JF, Friedlander BR and Ireland BK. Interpretation of low to moderate relative risks in environmental epidemiologic studies. Annual Review of Public Health 1994;15:179–201.

Allen BC, Crump KS and Shipp AM. Correlation between carcinogenic potency of chemical in animals and humans. Risk Analysis 1988;8:531–561. [comments by Hart R, Turturro A, Crouch E, Portier CJ, Silbergold E]

Annest JL, Pirkle JL, Makric D, Neese JW, Bayse DD and Kovac MG. Chronological trend in blood lead levels between 1976 and 1980. N Engl J Med 1983;308:1373–1377.

Armitage P and Doll R. Stochastic models for carcinogenesis. In: J. Neyman (eds) Proceedings of the Fourth Berkeley Symposium on Mathematical Statistics and Probability, 1961;4:19–38.

Armstrong BK, White E and Saracci R. Principles of Exposure Measurement. In: Epidemiology. Oxford: Oxford University Press, 1992.

Becher H and Wahrendorf. Variability of unit risk estimates under different statistical models and between different epidemiological data sets. In: Moolgavkar SH (eds) Scientific Issues in Quantitative Cancer Risk Assessment. Boston: Birhauser Pub., 1990.

Blair A and Stewart PA. Comments on the Sterling and Weikam Analysis of Data from the National Cancer Institute Formaldehyde Study. Am J Indust Med 1994;25:603–606.

Breslow NE, Lubin JH, Malek P and Langholz B. Multiplicative models and cohort analysis. J Am Stat Assoc 1983;78:1–12.

Centers for Disease Control. Guidelines for investigation of clusters of health events. Morbid Mortal Weekly Rep 1990;39(No. RR-11):1–22.

Checkoway H. Determining the hazards of workplace chemicals. Epidemiology 1993;4:91–92.

Cole P, Delzell E and Acquavella S. Exposure to butadiene and lymphatic and hematopoietic cancer. Epidemiology 1993;4:96–103.

Correa A, Stewart WF, Hsin-Chieh Y and Santos-Burogoa C. Exposure measurement case-control studies: reported methods and recommendations. Epidemiologic Reviews 1994;16(1):18–32.

Deane M, Swan S, Harrios JA, Epstein DM and Neutra RR. Adverse pregnancy outcomes in relation to waters consumption: A re-analysis of data from the original Santa Clara County study, California, 1980–1981. Epidemiology 1992;3:94–97.

Elcock M and Morgan RW. Update on artificial sweetners and bladder cancer. Reg Tox Pharm 1993;17: 35–43.

Environmental Protection Agency, "Draft Working Paper for Considering Draft Revisions to the EPA Guidelines for Cancer Risk Assessment", Washington DC, November 1992.

Environmental Protection Agency, "Guidelines for Carcinogen Risk Assessment", Federal Register, vol. 51, 24 September 1986, pp. 33992+.

Epidemiology Task Group. Guidelines for Good Epidemiology Practices for Occupational and Environmental Epidemiologic Research. Chemical Manufacturers Association, Washington DC, 1991.

Feldgoise D. Human Epidemiology Used in Quantifying Risk, Internal Report, Harvard Center for Risk Analysis, Boston, MA, October 1993.

Gold LS, Manley NB and Ames BN. Extrapolation of carcinogenicity between species: qualitative and quantitative factors. Risk Analysis 1992;12:579–588.

Graham JD et al. In Search of Safety, 1988.

Harvard Center for Risk Analysis. Risk Assessment in the Federal Government: Questions and Answers, Harvard School of Public Health, Boston, MA, October 1993.

Harvard Center for Risk Analysis. A Historical Perspective in Risk Assessment in the Federal Government, Harvard School of Public Health, Boston, MA, March 1994.

Hawkins NC. Conservatism in maximally exposed individual predictive exposure assessments: a first-Cut analysis. Regul Toxicol Pharmacol 1991;14:107–117.

Hill AB. The environment and disease: association or causation. Proc R Soc Med 1965;58:295–300.

Industrial Union Department, AFL-CIO v. American Petroleum Institute, 448 U.S. Supreme Court, 1980;607.

International Program on Chemical Safety, United Nations Environment Programme. Report of IPCS Discussions on Deriving Guidance Values for Health-Based Exposure Limits, World Health Organization, Geneva, 1992.

Kaldor J. The role of epidemiological observation in elucidating the mechanisms of carcinogenesis. In: Vaino H, Magee P, McGregor D, McMichael AJ (eds) Mechanisms of Carcinogenesis: Risk Identification. IARC Scientific Publications No. 116, International Agency for Research on Cancer, Lyon, 1992.

Katz EA, Shaw GM and Shaffer DM. Exposure assessment in epidemiologic studies of birth defects by industrial hygiene review of material interviews. Am J Indust Med 1994;26:1–11.

Lagakos SW, Wessen BI and Zelem M. An analysis of contaminated well water and health effects in Woburn Massachusetts. J Am Stat Assoc 1986;81:583–596.

Last JM (eds). A Dictionary of Epidemiology. Oxford: Oxford University Press, 1988.

Lave LB, Ennever F, Rosenkrantz HS and Omenn GS. Information value of the rodent bioessay. Nature 1988;336:631–633.

14

Lave L et al. 1988.

Layard MW and Silvers A. Epidemiology in environmental risk assessment. In: Paustenbach DJ (ed) Environmental and Occupational Risk Assessment: A Textbook of Case Studies. Chapter 3. New York: John Wiley and Sons, 1989.

Leung HJ and Paustenbach DJ. Assessing health risks in the workplace: a study of 2,3,7,8-tetra-chlorodibenze-p-dioxin. In: Paustenbach DJ (eds) The Risk Assessment of Environmental and Human Health Hazards: A Textbook of Case Studies. Chapter 20. John Wiley and Sons, New York, NY, 1989.

Matanowski GM and Santos-Burgoa C. Butadiene and lymphatic and hematopoietic cancer [Letter]. Epidemiology 1994;5:261—263.

Monson R. Occupational Epidemiology, Second Edition, CRC Press, Boca Raton, FA, 1990.

Omenn GS. The role of environmental epidemiology in public policy. Annals of Epidemiology 1993;3:319—322.

Parle RM. Butadiene epidemiology reinterpreted, again [letter]. Epidemiology 1993;4:559—560.

Parkin DM, Wagner G and Muir CS (eds). The Role of the Registry in Cancer Control. IARC Scientific Publications No 66, International Agency for Research on Cancer, Lyon, 1985.

Paustenbach DJ, Price PS, Ollison W, Blank C, Jernigan JD, Bass RD and Peterson HD. Revaluation of benzene exposure for the Pliofilm (Rubberworker) Cohort (1936—1976). Tox Environ Health 1992;6:177—231.

Rappaport SM and Smith JJ (eds). Exposure Assessment for Epidemiology and Hazard Control. Lewis Publishers, Chelsea, MI, 1991.

Rodericks J. Calculated Risks, Cambridge University Press, New York, NY, 1992.

Samet T (eds). Assessing Low-Risk Agents for Lung Cancer: Methodological Aspects. Int J Epidemiol 1990;19(1).

Sterling TD and Weinkam JJ. Mortality from respiratory cancers (including lung cancer) among workers employed in formaldehyde industries, Am J Indust Med 1994;25:593—602.

Wald NJ and Doll R (eds). Interpretation of negative epidemiological evidence for carcinogenicity. IARC Scientific Publications No. 65, International Agency for Research on Cancer, Lyon, 1985.

Whittemore A. Epidemiology in risk assessment for regulatory policy. J Chronic Dis 1986;39:1157—1168.

©1995 Elsevier Science B.V. All rights reserved.
The Role of Epidemiology in Regulatory Risk Assessment
J.D. Graham, editor.

Scientific criteria for the use of epidemiologic data in risk assessment

Genevieve Matanoski
School of Hygiene and Public Health, The Johns Hopkins University, Baltimore, Maryland, USA

Key words: assessment, decision, dose-response, epidemiology, hazard, regulation, risk.

Introduction

The early studies of environmental risks from air pollution made extensive use of human data to determine potential effects. As the Environmental Protection Agency first started business in December 1970, there were no rules for the methods of assessing risks (Ruckelshaus). Then gradually in its development, EPA established the methods of quantitative risk assessment as we know it today and it has become an accepted part of the regulatory decision process (Goldstein, 1988). The components of the assessment follow guidelines established within the agency and recommended by the National Research Council (EPA, 1983; NAS, 1983). The components of the process include hazard identification, dose-response estimation, exposure assessment and risk characterization. Many of the chemicals reviewed under this process can be regulated without any data to directly suggest that the agent is a human carcinogen. Federal agencies can regulate a compound on the basis of simple long-term studies showing cancer in multiple organs in both sexes in multiple species and they are willing to accept these data to set mandates without using any human data. This is a far cry from the original studies of air pollution and the risks on human health. Why the change? Is it because cancer is the endpoint of primary interest in risk assessment at present and this chronic effect of exposure may be difficult to determine in humans? Is it that the quantitative response assessment is difficult to develop from human data? Is it that human data are not subject to the same control on confounding variables such as other exposures or susceptibility as are possible in laboratory animals and so are always subject to more controversy than animal data?

The current discussion will examine the use of epidemiological or nonexperimental human data as a source of information for risk assessment. It will examine the pros

---

Address for correspondence: Genevieve Matanoski, Professor of Epidemiology, School of Hygiene and Public Health, The Johns Hopkins University, 624 North Broadway, Room 280, Baltimore, MD 21205, USA. Tel.: +1-410–955–8183. Fax: +1-410–276–0290.

and cons of using the data and the possible situations under which they are useful. The paper will also examine the role, if any, of molecular epidemiology and biomarkers in risk assessment and its essential role in assessments when outcomes other than cancer are involved.

Role of epidemiology in risk assessment

The primary advantage of epidemiologic data is obvious. The risks are assessed in the population of interest, the human. The physiologic characteristics are those of interest. While there may be variations in humans, basic features are similar. The individual variations in characteristics such as enzymatic capabilities to process certain chemicals would still be less variable than would be the major variations across species. One constant controversy facing regulatory agencies, the question of whether mice are like men, would be eliminated.

The second important consideration is that the range of diseases which may be affected by an agent can be expanded. However difficult it may be to examine cancers in rodents and apply the data to humans, determination of effects that might impact on several systems such as respiratory, neurologic, cardiac and immunologic may be even more difficult to examine in nonhuman species. Impacts of exposures on reasoning capabilities, asthma, arteriosclerotic or hypertensive changes in heart and blood vessel may be impossible to adequately measure in populations which have widely discrepant physiology or different related variables as diet or in whom the outcome cannot be measured. Therefore, with a growing demand to examine outcomes of toxic exposures beyond cancer or even reproductive abnormalities, the human will need to be the source of risk assessment data. Use of direct experimentation is generally impossible, so epidemiologic data must be collected for populations of interest.

A final point to consider is that epidemiologic data are collected under exposure conditions and at levels that are directly relevant to the true human situation (Shore, 1992). Thus, even high to low dose extrapolations from a work setting to the general population occur over a range of magnitude which is smaller than that used in animal studies.

The major disadvantage of epidemiologic data appears to lie in the fact that the data are subject to more controversy. Data on high exposures generally come from occupational settings and questions arise whether this natural experiment applies to the general population (Matanoski, 1988). The susceptibility of populations in various settings may differ from the total US. The presence of multiple hazards may be difficult to sort out in terms of which agents actually caused the risk. The conditions under which the exposure takes place as in industrial settings may be different than that which occurs in the home. For example, intake of air under conditions of heavy exertion in a working environment may differ from that of activities in the home.

The final example suggests the most serious problem which has restricted use of epidemiologic data in risk assessment is the problem of determining exposure and dose-response. Epidemiologic data has no difficulty identifying disease which is acute and follows directly from a recent exposure. In the case of studies of asthma in the indoor environment, there may be some questions about the factors which are related to the susceptibility of the subject, but exposure to even minute quantities of the sensitizing agent can prompt immediate response which can be measured. Even single exposures to a hazard and a delayed event such as cancer can be measured in a population and used for risk assessment without much controversy. For example, the data from the atomic bomb exposure and the subsequent Japanese survivor cancer experience are a major source for estimating risks from radiation. However, diseases with long latency and repeated exposures in the population have created problems in determining exposures and relating outcomes to the exposure. Part of the problem arises from the fact that epidemiology is not focused on determining the permissible dose. The emphasis has been on trying to decide whether it is more likely than not that an agent causes a specific outcome of interest. Then based on epidemiologist's experience with infectious agents and cigarette smoke, the aim of the studies was to eliminate the cause. Dose-response was simply a tool to establishing probable causation, not a means to develop a standard of exposure (Matanoski, 1988; Shore, 1992). Even the models which have been used to establish risk have been those that assume a constant multiple of risk over all doses. The analysis of the epidemiologic data is often not detailed enough to provide the needed information regarding the appropriate dose-response model.

Basic criteria for using epidemiologic data

Risk assessment using animal data moved forward rapidly following the establishment of standards regarding the methods of assessing hazard identification and dose-response. The epidemiologists have resisted attempts to set criteria for evaluating epidemiologic studies while gradually imposing standards through peer review in journals and in research proposal evaluation. However, over the past several years, weight-of-evidence approaches to data from epidemiologic studies has gradually developed more in the area of therapy than in the area of risk. We have utilized the results from several observational epidemiologic studies to make decisions regarding potential benefits from postmenopausal estrogen therapy. While the data still may have problems delineating effective dose, approximate levels can be determined. The information might be improved with further thought. The time is appropriated to begin to consider how epidemiologic data can be combined to use in risk assessment.

Several criteria for appropriate collection of epidemiologic data apply to all good studies. The study design and the collection of information must be sound. No study is perfect so the judgement must be made whether any of the flaws could seriously influence results. A simple recitation of the litany of the potential variables that cannot be addressed in any study is not useful. The question is whether any of the flaws could change the conclusion particularly if that conclusion has been reached using multiple studies with possible different constraints. Any possible bias in the studies should be identified since this could influence results. The outcomes and the evaluation must be carefully considered. Confirmation of the disease or direct examination of individuals may be needed in some cases. The populations must be large enough and followed long enough to anticipate finding sufficient numbers of events for analysis.

The most important consideration which has restrained the use of epidemiologic studies for risk assessment has been the lack of usable information on dose. In the analysis of dose, the handling of repetitive exposures and the biologic responses to such challenges as well as their relationship to the final outcomes need to be considered. Many of the exposures from which risks are assessed arise in occupational settings. While the exposures and follow-up of these populations in terms of assessing exposure is more feasible than most household exposures, these populations have little available information on personal and lifestyle characteristics. Efforts to determine exposures retrospectively for occupational risk studies are still in their infancy. The methods of estimating exposures over long times, with repeated doses during those periods and variation and uncertainty in the methods used to determine exposures have not been totally evaluated in terms of how these factors will influence risk assessment. The emphasis initially was to determine what the exposure was for each individual in a population. However, that is not necessary for the epidemiology study. Samples of the populations are adequate and relative exposure levels may be sufficient. Further consideration must be given to what level of detail is necessary and how to use the measures to predict the true exposure. Biologic information on how to transform the environmental exposures to actual dose then become important. Individuals because of their personal biologic profile or their activities within the exposure situation can alter the physiologically effective dose.

Regardless of the difficulty in obtaining exposure information and the uncertainty in the results, if we are to use human information for risk assessment then we must move beyond classifying individuals by "ever/never" exposed to obtain some detail regarding exposure. In this endeavor, information on duration of exposure alone is not enough but at a minimum data on duration plus intensity is needed. An examination of the variation in the data, reasons for the variation and the points which produce uncertainty in some of data could lead to further refinement of the dose-response assessment. While this level of detail will not be attempted for every agent to which individuals may be exposed, it could be reserved for those where an effect is suspected. The important step may not be to look at all the possible sources of incomplete information and try to fill in the gaps, but to examine the data to determine to which of the problems is the outcome of the dose-response analysis most sensitive.

Analysis of epidemiologic data might benefit by adding a question of "what if" to answer the concerns about whether the estimates that are derived are more probable than not and are not likely to vary beyond a certain range of values. This then allows for us to evaluate the strength of the epidemiologic observations. It also permits us to identify the uncertainties in the analysis and identify the assumptions in the analysis. This means that the data must be analyzed using different assumptions in regard to models, standard errors and other variables to determine whether different conclusions regarding risks may be appropriate or unlikely. The importance of identifying a specific overtly defined set of assumptions which are tested in the risk assessments means that there is a repeatable mathematical statement which can describe all assumptions.

The guidelines for use of epidemiologic data are difficult to establish for all diseases but this also is true for animal data. Cancer guidelines for toxicological experiments were successful because they were established primarily on the basis that cancer results from direct damage to DNA and that an increase in the cumulative dose of the carcinogen should result in increased probability of damage to the genetic material of the cells in the target organ. However, even cancer effects are not that simple in either animals or humans. Certainly when we move to other effects, such as reproductive and neurologic, the exposures and the effects have a much more complicated biologic interaction. Pharmacokinetic actions of the chemicals on various organ systems becomes important since the effects may not be one which is directly targeted to the organ interest. Timing of the exposure in developing fetuses and in brain tissue of the fetus and newborn will be more important than total dose of the toxicant. The point is that the biologic consideration of the method of developing disease and the pharmacokinetic action of the agent on the tissue must be studied more extensively in order to identify dose-response relationships for the many agents which are not directly genotoxic and may cause diseases other than cancer.

Risk assessments generally have accounted for differential susceptibility in the population by adding a "protective factor" to the dose-response measure. Yet, in many situations there are known differences in response related to certain basic characteristics of the population. Some of the common characteristics we suspect alter risk would be age especially in the extremes as fetuses, children, the elderly. Persons with other chronic diseases may respond differently, especially if they are on medication. The data from the pharmaceutical literature would suggest that people's responses differ by race and sex as well. The epidemiologic data used for iden- tification of hazards may include some of these individuals in the risk estimate but not usually children and elderly. New consideration must be given as to how one will account for the differences in risk based on personal characteristics in the evaluation of the risk assessment. This is a growing issue as the research community continues to develop methods of detecting differences in risk profiles of individuals. The future may hold a promise of being able to characterize each individual for their personal risk. We would not need to use general characteristics such as age, race and sex then to determine risk groups. The question is what the regulator must do to protect the health of the individual as we learn how to characterize risk more specifically on a personal basis.

The discussion has focused on the role of epidemiology and criteria for its use in the first two phases of risk assessment — hazard identification and dose-response. However, epidemiology also plays a role in identification of exposure in the general population and in characterization of the population at risk. Both of these activities estimate the potential exposure of populations. In such activities, the regulatory agencies have frequently ignored the importance of human variation and neglected to account for this in decisions on exposure assessment and risk characterization. The models which assess residential exposure as if it is a constant for 70 years are not realistic and require further evaluation for the impact of population mobility. The lack of attention to such epidemiologic principles as the simultaneous examination of all routes of exposure rather than separate assessments are important refinements to include in human models. Competing risks in terms of assessing impact of a carcinogen and comorbidities from other toxic exposures could change the impact of a chemical on populations.

New directions to improve use

The field of molecular epidemiology is expanding the horizons for potential use of epidemiologic data in the future. The presence of a carcinogen even in the past may leave a marker on the genome of cells which changes the individual risks for the future (Brashi, 1992). The studies of humans are indicating more about the basic hereditary characteristics of the person which may change his/her susceptibility (Wei et al., 1994). The pharmacokinetics of the action of a toxic in the human as opposed to the animal may require a different evaluation than the direct extrapolation from animal to man. The methods for bringing some of these new biologic and epidemiologic data into use in risk assessment have not been described.

Imperative for the future

Epidemiology must become a major tool in quantitative risk assessment. However, until there are accepted scientific criteria for utilizing the data, it will continue to be considered a field for controversy. Industry and the regulators will tend to embrace opposing studies as warranting sole consideration. Arguments will arise as to whether the confounding factors have been taken into account. Decisions regarding significance of the findings and appropriateness of selected controls will continue to dominate the discussion. Science and especially epidemiology does not always produce unequivocal results. Data are subject to various interpretations. Therefore, it is appropriate to review the criteria for appropriate interpretation of epidemiologic studies and to help the risk assessors evaluate human data if we expect them to utilize such data for environmental protection.

References

Brashi DE, Rudolf JA, Simon JA, Lin A, McKenna GJ, Baden HP, Halperin AJ and Ponten J. A role for sunlight in skin cancer. UV-induced p53 mutations in squamous cell carcinoma. Proc Natl Acad Sci USA 1991;88:10124–10128.

Goldstein BD. The scientific basis for policy decision. In: Gordis L (ed) Epidemiology and Health Risk Assessment (Chapter 2), New York: Oxford University Press, 1988.

National Academy of Sciences Commitee on the Institutional Means for Assessment of Risks to Public Health, 1983. Risk Assessment in the Federal Government: Managing the Process. Washington DC: National Academy Press.

Ruckelshaus WD. U.S. EPA Oral History. Interview-1. Washington DC. SAIC Inc. VA, Jan, 1993.

Shore RE, Iyer V, Altshuler B and Pasternack BS. Use of human data in quantitative risk assessment of carcinogens: impact on epidemiologic practice and the regulatory process. Reg Toxicol Pharmacol 1992;15:180–221.

Wei Q, Matanoski GM, Farmer ER, Hedayati MA and Grossman L. DNA repair and aging in basal cell carcinoma: a molecular epidemiology study. Proc Natl Acad Sci USA 1993;90:1614–1618.

©1995 Elsevier Science B.V. All rights reserved.
The Role of Epidemiology in Regulatory Risk Assessment
J.D. Graham, editor.

Scientific criteria for the use of epidemiology data in risk assessment: comment

Gregory G. Bond

Global Director of Product Stewardship, The Dow Chemical Company, Chemicals, Performance Products and Hydrocarbons

Abstract. This article was prepared for presentation at the federal focus conference, "the proper role of epidemiology in regulatory risk assessment", October 13–14, 1994, Lansdowne Conference Center, Lansdowne, Virginia.

Key words: assessment, criteria, epidemiology, hypothesis-generating, hypothesis-testing, meta-analysis, risk.

Introduction

Let me begin by complimenting Dr Matanoski on her very thoughtful review of criteria for the use of epidemiology data in risk assessment (Matanoski, 1994). She correctly notes that epidemiologists have generally resisted attempts to set criteria for evaluating studies, instead relying on peer review of grant applications and publications. However, as Graham (1994) has shown, this is not working, and it is now essential for epidemiologists to provide formal guidance to regulators and other decision-makers. This is not a new revelation. Several thought leaders in the field of epidemiology have previously suggested the need for such guidance (Gordis, 1988; Rothman, 1993), but for some reason it has not been forthcoming. Hopefully, this conference will provide the needed stimulus.

A distinction will be drawn in this paper between criteria for evaluating the quality of data from individual epidemiologic studies and criteria for assessing a body of epidemiologic evidence for risk assessment purposes. In doing so, focus will be directed at four items which Dr. Matanoski mentioned only briefly or did not discuss, namely: the need to include all of the available high quality evidence in risk assessments; criteria for evaluating the quality of epidemiologic research, including the need for "Good Epidemiology Practices", an ongoing controversy regarding the relative weight that should be accorded hypothesis-generating vs. hypothesis-testing research; and finally, some thoughts on dealing with discordant results, including a

Address for correspondence: Gregory G. Bond, PhD, MPH. Health and Environmental Sciences, Dow Chemical Company, 1803 Building, Midland, MI 48674, USA. Tel.: +1-517-636-9063. Fax: +1-517-636-1875.

brief discussion of meta-analysis. Some areas where epidemiologists still need to develop consensus will be highlighted.

Increasing use of epidemiology data in risk assessments

Both Graham (1994) and Matanoski (1994) predict an increase in the use of epidemiological evidence for regulatory risk assessment. This may very well occur; however, the U.S. Environmental Protection Agency (EPA) and other regulatory agencies currently appear more than willing to regulate agents based on rodent data alone. Perhaps most notable in this regard is the EPA's recently released draft reassessment of dioxin and dioxin-like compounds (U.S. EPA, 1994) which, in addition to expressing traditional concerns about cancer, cites new evidence of effects on reproductive behavior and the immune system based almost exclusively on data from rodent studies. The EPA's tendency to undervalue near-null epidemiological evidence acts as an unintended disincentive for sponsorship of epidemiological research. This situation is unfortunate and needs to be reversed so that an optimal amount of quality epidemiological data are available for risk assessment purposes.

Criteria for evaluating the quality of epidemiology studies

It appears that epidemiologists and risk assessors are arriving at a consensus that all good quality epidemiological data, regardless of whether it is positive or near null, should be considered in hazard identification (Doll, 1985; Ahlbom, 1990). In a recent review article, Shore et al. (1992) stated that "Risk assessment should be viewed as a measurement process in which the magnitude of effects (per unit dose) are estimated, then good quality negative (null) evidence is just as valid as positive evidence and should be accorded appropriate weight in the risk assessment process." However, this then begs the question, "What constitutes good quality evidence?". For the purposes of this paper, good quality evidence will be defined as having been derived from good quality epidemiological research.

Epidemiological research is usually judged according to several criteria:
— study design;
— data quality;
— avoidance or control of technical biases, typically described as selection, misclassification (or information), and confounding;
— appropriate analysis methods;
— sound data presentation.

With few exceptions, most of the epidemiological research which has relevance for risk assessment will have been derived from either case control or historical cohort study designs. All other things being equal, cohort studies are generally considered to provide stronger evidence than case-control studies, because they are less prone to technical biases introduced by sampling and data collection and have superior quantitative estimates of exposure (Morgenstern and Thomas, 1993). In general then, evidence from cohort studies should be given greater weight than evidence from case-control studies.

Several points need to be made about data quality. Obviously, the underlying data needs to be sound and well-documented. The EPA (TSCA, 1989; FIFRA, 1989) have indicated their desire to audit epidemiological data for quality, yet few guidelines for such audits exist (OMB, 1988). Several years ago, a Chemical Manufacturers Association Task Force drafted "Good Epidemiology Practices" or GEPs (CMA, 1991) in an attempt to fill this void. Analogous to Good Laboratory Practices or GLPs which exist to guide toxicological research, the GEPs outline guidance for practices and procedures that should be considered in order to help ensure the quality and integrity of data used in epidemiological research and to provide adequate documentation of the research methods. It is difficult to know precisely how widely these guidelines are practiced, but if references to them in journal publications are any indication, it must be fairly rare. This is unfortunate for, if they are to be used in risk assessment, epidemiological data must be subject to the same level of quality control as toxicological data. This should be true regardless of who sponsors or conducts the research.

As Matanoski (1994) noted, exposure estimates are typically the "Achilles-heel" of occupational and environmental epidemiology, and it is because of poorly characterized and documented exposures that epidemiological findings have not been used more often in risk assessment. Others (Checkoway et al., 1989; Shore et al., 1992) have written extensively on this subject, so it will not be dealt with in any great detail here. It is sufficient to say that this is an area of increase focus by teams of investigators including epidemiologists, industrial hygienists, chemists and molecular biologists. With the advent of more extensive exposure monitoring in the workplace during the 1970s, and the future promise of biomarkers, opportunities to use good quality exposure estimates should increase.

Studies need to be directed at large groups with high enough exposures to provide sufficient statistical power to make near null results persuasive. Likewise, the timing of exposures in relation to the observation period must be relevant. For studies of reproductive events, exposures must have occurred shortly before or during critical stages of fetal development. For studies of cancer, study subjects need to have been followed for a sufficient length of time after exposure for latent periods to be expressed. Obviously, evidence of a dose-response in the relation between exposure and disease greatly improves the strength of the evidence.

Much has been written about selection, misclassification and confounding bias (Morgenstern and Thomas, 1993), and as Matanoski has noted, it is not enough to simply list them — an effort needs to be made to examine the data to determine the approximate magnitude and the direction of any impact. Strong associations, i.e., generally speaking, relative risk estimates above two, are less likely to be the result of technical biases. Complicating matters, however, is the reality that many of the environmental risk factors now being evaluated are likely to be only weakly associated with disease so that technical biases remain an alternative explanation for the results.

In the area of data analysis, tremendous strides have been made to develop sophisticated statistical analysis tools and they are easily accessible to most epidemiologists. While this has allowed very efficient use of complex data sets, it has also led to problems in some instances. An issue that is especially troublesome is that of multiple comparisons. Since data are typically available for a large number of diseases and/or exposures, epidemiologists often feel obliged to analyze all possible permutations. The probability of obtaining at least one statistically significant result by chance becomes quite high as the number of statistical comparisons increases. Epidemiologists are frequently reluctant to employ corrections for multiple comparisons, preferring instead to rely on professional judgment in making interpretations. This often leads to controversy and confusion for risk assessors, and thus it is an issue that needs resolution.

Another analysis issue involves an ongoing debate among epidemiologists concerning whether or not findings derived from hypothesis-generating studies need to be given less weight than those from hypothesis testing studies (Gordis, 1988; Skrabanek, 1994; Savitz, 1994). The former have been referred to variously as "fishing expeditions" or "black box" epidemiology. Advocates of hypothesis-generating research argue that it has been the source of the most important findings thus far, and that there is no logical link between the quality of the evidence derived from such research and prior evidence of a causal association from other types of research. Its detractors argue for more biological underpinnings for epidemiological research and greater caution in interpreting findings in the absence of a biologically plausible, prior hypothesis. Doll (1984) has gone so far as to suggest that when subsequent hypothesis-testing research has been done, the original hypothesis-generating findings should be excluded from the risk assessment.

A related issue deals with what Shore et al. (1992) have referred to as indiscriminate analysis of subgroups. This amounts to an investigator torturing the data set until it "squeals the truth". This is relevant to our current discussion because Matanoski has justifiably argued for evaluation of multiple exposure models, i.e., many subgroups. Such evaluations, particularly dose-response analyses, are critical as they increase the statistical power of the study and decrease the potential for false negative results. However, in light of the foregoing discussion of the problems of multiple comparisons and biological plausibility, it seems reasonable to recommend that some caution be taken in interpreting the findings from evaluations of multiple subgroups.

Due to the prevalence of environmental exposures and particular diseases of interest, quite low in the population, many epidemiology studies have low statistical power. This has typically been a criticism of near null findings, i.e., a real increase risk was missed because the sample size was too small. But low statistical power also has implications for studies which purport to show an effect. Land (1981) has shown that if a study has low power and a positive result is found, the size of the risk will almost surely be overestimated and potentially by a large amount. This provides an additional reason to be cautious when interpreting the results of a single study which shows an association.

Criteria for use of epidemiological data in risk assessment

The foregoing discussion has focused solely on criteria for evaluating epidemiological data derived from individual studies. A distinction has purposely been drawn between those criteria and the criteria used to evaluate evidence from multiple studies for two reasons:
— the data from a single study should first be judged on their own merits without considering other evidence;
— only data that are judged to be of sufficiently high quality should be considered for use in regulatory risk assessments.

It is almost never the case that a single epidemiology study alone is sufficient to establish a cause and effect relationship between an exposure and disease. Instead, an association must be repeatedly observed by different investigators in different places, circumstances and times. An association is further strengthened if there is experimental support for it from toxicological studies. In such instances when the human and animal data are concordant, a regulator could feel quite confident about using all of the data for risk assessment purposes. Yet, scenarios wherein all of the data are concordant are extremely rare. More often, the evidence is conflicting and the task of the regulator is quite complex.

Doll (1985) has suggested that, when the data are discordant, a weight of the evidence approach employing all of the high quality data should be used. When there is extensive, high quality human evidence, regardless of whether it is positive or near null, it should be given greater weight than rodent toxicology data of doubtful generality (Shore et al., 1992). Even when the human data are not extensive, the upper bound of the 95% confidence intervals can provide a useful plausibility check on a quantitative risk assessment derived solely from rodent data.

In some instances, the epidemiology data may be quite extensive, but the various risk estimates from the individual studies are inconsistent. Such situations are fraught with controversy. More frequently, meta-analysis is being applied in an attempt to derive more precise and valid risk estimates (Greenland, 1987). This technique remains under development, and there are many issues yet to be resolved, including questions as to how to effectively deal with publication bias (i.e., a tendency for near null results to be less often published than positive results), and whether and how to weight individual studies based on their quality. Even so, meta-analysis offers some promise for improving the contribution epidemiology can make to risk assessment.

Conclusion

Opportunities exist to increase the use of epidemiology to improve quantitative risk assessment. To realize them, epidemiologists must be willing to provide regulators with greater guidance for assessing the quality of individual studies and for resolving discordant results among and between epidemiological and toxicological research. Expanding on the paper of Matanoski (1994), this paper has outlined some practical

28

guidance which could be helpful. Yet, it has also identified some areas where controversy among epidemiologists remains. It is imperative that epidemiologists work together among themselves and with toxicologists, statisticians and risk assessors to analyze case studies to develop practical solutions for dealing with the remaining issues.

References

Ahlbom A, Axelson O, Hansen E et al. Interpretation of "negative" studies in occupational epidemiology. Scand J Work Environ Health 1990;16:153—157.

Checkoway H, Pearce N, Crawford-Brown D. Research Methods in Occupational Epidemiology. New York: Oxford University Press, 1989.

Chemical Manufacturers Association. Guidelines for Good Epidemiology Practices for Occupational and Environmental Epidemiologic Research. CMA, Washington, DC, 1991.

Doll R. Occupational cancer: problems in interpreting human evidence. Ann Occup Hyg 1984;28:291—305.

Doll R. Purpose of symposium. In: Wald NJ and Doll R (eds) Interpretation of Negative Epidemiological Evidence for Carcinogenicity. Lyon: International Agency for Research on Cancer, 1985;3—10.

Federal Insecticide, Fungicide, and Rodenticide Act (FIFRA). Good Laboratory Practice Standards. 54 FED. REG. 34052, August 17, 1989.

Gordis L. Challenges to epidemiology in the next decade. Am J Epidemiol 1988;128:1—9.

Graham J.D. Epidemiology and risk assessment: they aren't antonyms. Presented at the Federal Focus Conference, "The Proper Role of Epidemiology in Regulatory Risk Assessment", Lansdowne, MD, October 13—14, 1994.

Greenland S. Quantitative methods in the review of epidemiologic literature. Epidemiol Rev 1987;9:1—30.

Land C. Statistical limitations in relation to sample size. Environ Health Perspect 1981;42:15—21.

Matanoski G. Scientific criteria for the use of epidemiologic data in risk assessment. Presented at the Federal Focus Conference, "The Proper Role of Epidemiology in Regulatory Risk Assessment", Lansdowne, MD, October 13—14, 1994.

Morgenstern H, Thomas D. Principles of study design in environmental epidemiology. Environ Health Perspect 1993;101(suppl 4):23—38.

Office of Management and Budget (OMB). Guidelines for Federal Statistical Activities. 53 FED. REG. 1542, January 20, 1988.

Rothman KJ. Methodologic frontiers in environmental epidemiology. Environ Health Perspect 1993;101 (Suppl 4):19—21.

Savitz DA. In defense of black box epidemiology. Epidemiology 1994;5:550—552.

Skrabanek P. The emptiness of the black box. Epidemiology 1994;5:553—555.

Shore RE, Iyer V, Altshuler B, Pasternack B. Use of human data in quantitative risk assessment of carcinogens: impact on epidemiologic practice and the regulatory process. Regulatory Toxicol Pharmacol 1992;15:180—221.

Toxic Substances Control Act (TSCA). Good Laboratory Practice Standards. 54 FED. REG. 34034, August 17, 1989.

U.S. EPA. Draft health assessment document for 2,3,7,8-tetrachlorodibenzo-p-dioxin (TCDD) and related compounds, Volumes I, II, and III, EPA/600/BP—92/001a, 001b, 001c. Washington, DC, 1994.

©1995 Elsevier Science B.V. All rights reserved.
The Role of Epidemiology in Regulatory Risk Assessment
J.D. Graham, editor.

Biases introduced by confounding and imperfect retrospective and prospective exposure assessments

Alvan R. Feinstein

Sterling Professor of Medicine and Epidemiology, Yale University School of Medicine, New Haven, Connecticut, USA

Key words: bias, confounding, methodology, rate ratios, reproducibility, risk, standards, variables.

The epidemiologic appraisal of risk factors is a cause-effect analysis in which the "risk factor" is an exposure that is believed to cause or promote development of a particular disease. The exposure is usually an external entity — such as atmospheric pollution, diet, or smoking — but can also be a person's internal biologic attribute, such as sex or family history.

The "gold-standard" method of research for cause-effect analysis in human disease is the experiment called a *randomized trial*. During the past few decades, such trials have commonly been used to evaluate the cause-effect benefits of therapeutic agents, but randomized trials are seldom possible when the agent is believed to be a noxious risk factor. Many people would regard the trial as unethical if it is done because the agent is suspected of doing harm rather than good; and even if the ethical issue can be rationalized, the trial would seldom be feasible. Too few people, if prepared for a suitably informed consent, would volunteer to participate.

Consequently, data about risk factors seldom come from randomized trials; and epidemiologists have become accustomed to doing research with observational evidence, obtained and analyzed in nonexperimental designs that substitute for the desired trial that could not be done. The observational evidence is obtained for groups of people whose investigated events occurred in the natural circumstances of daily life.

The main point I want to make in this discussion, is that although a randomized trial contains many scientific principles beyond the randomized assignment itself, those principles are usually ignored or abandoned in many — perhaps most — epidemiologic studies of risk factors for the cancers, infarctions, atherosclerosis and other noninfectious diseases that have major societal importance. Instead, the epidemiologists tend to rely on mathematical models and assumptions that may have all the majesty of elegant (and sometimes mysterious) statistics, while lacking many of the basic principles of scientific research (Feinstein, 1988, 1989).

Address for correspondence: Alvan R. Feinstein, Clinical Epidemiology Unit, 333 Cedar Street, Yale University School of Medicine, New Haven, CT 06510, USA. Tel.: +1-203-785-5177. Fax: +1-203-785-4146.

In the usual statistical report about an epidemiologic risk factor, a particular disease is associated with a particular exposure; and the results are usually cited as risk ratios for the occurrence rates of disease in the exposed vs. nonexposed groups. To avoid the threat of clarity, these ratios are also called by various other names, such as relative risks, and rate ratios. In the commonly used case-control studies, in which risk ratios cannot be determined, the comparative results are usually expressed as an odds ratio, which can mathematically approximate a risk ratio, if the disease has a low rate of occurrence (such as below .01) *and* if the case-control results suitably represent the preceding cause-effect pathway.

Statistical approaches to confounding

The idea of a cause-effect pathway, however, is itself often rejected or disdained by prominent statistical epidemiologists (Cornfield, 1954; Greenland and Morganstern, 1988; Miettinen, 1988; Rothman, 1986) who often argue that all cause-effect relationships are associations, and that little or no attention need be given to the sequence and time direction in which the actual events occurred. With this belief, everything can be analyzed as a statistical association between the two main variables for outcome and exposure; and all other phenomena become regarded as covariates to be "adjusted" with diverse forms of matching, stratification, or (most commonly) multivariable analysis.

The main reason for the adjustments, is to avoid or repair an entity called *confounding*, which is difficult to define, but is something that fouls up the statistical results, leading to distortions or misleading conclusions. For example, suppose statistics show that graduates of Ivy-League colleges have higher incomes and net worth in later life than graduates of other schools. The conclusion that an Ivy-League education leads to financial benefits in later life would be confounded by the generally more favorable familial and socio-economic conditions of the Ivy-League students before college begins. They may be starting out with more money, and may be given more along the way.

In the absence of attention to a scientific pathway, however, *confounding* is left without a specific source. It then becomes something like an early 19th century *miasma*, which was a nonspecific vapor that did evil things, but is not otherwise identified (Feinstein, 1985). Without a scientific strategy to guide the search, the customary statistical approach to confounding is to round up a set of available suspects: age, sex, occupation, height, weight, smoking, dietary habits, "lifestyle", and almost anything else for which data have been collected, beyond the main information about the suspected exposure and disease. In a multivariable analysis of the relationship between the alleged exposure and the suspected disease, the additional data become covariates that presumably adjust the results for "confounding".

Pathways of cause-effect events

For investigators who want to think about scientific biology rather than mathematical models, however, the phenomena of a cause-effect relationship do not occur merely as random events. Instead, the scientific reasoning for a cause-effect pathway begins with an entity that is constantly neglected or inadequately described in most statistical appraisals. This entity, to which I shall return again shortly, is the baseline state of the persons who become exposed or nonexposed. From their baseline state, they then undergo or decide to receive the exposure (or nonexposure), which can be performed with many accompanying phenomena that might be called coexposures. After a period of time during which the exposure and its coexposures may have continued or stopped, the persons are then found or not found to have the disease that is the focus of the research. At this phase in the sequence of events, however, the people are still statistically unremarkable. They do not achieve statistical recognition and become the subjects of research until something happens to transfer them from their anonymous state of natural existence into their mathematical immortality as units in a collected set of research data.

None of these movements from one location to another in the cause-effect pathway takes place randomly, and each movement can be accompanied by specific biases that produce confounding.

Susceptibility bias

In susceptibility bias, the persons who become exposed are prognostically more likely to develop the outcome event than those who are not exposed. The classical clinical example of susceptibility bias occurs in the therapy of cancer. Surgical treatment is generally reserved for "operable" patients, who usually have localized cancers *and* no major comorbid diseases. The "inoperable" patients, who have metastatic cancer and/or major comorbidity, are usually denied surgery and sent to receive radiotherapy or chemotherapy. These two groups of patients have strikingly different prognoses; and the "operable" group will have much better survival even if the surgery is not done. Nevertheless, survival rates are constantly compared for surgical vs. nonsurgical therapy, without regard to the confounding distortions of susceptibility bias.

In epidemiologic research for risk factors, susceptibility bias is not easy to illustrate, mainly because the investigators have seldom looked for it and collected satisfactory data. For example, many doctors and patients know that the best general way to have a long life span is to choose long-lived parents and other ancestors. Nevertheless, even though the data are easy to acquire, parental longevity is almost never recorded or analyzed in epidemiologic research. Suppose, however, that people with short-lived parents, suspecting that their own lives may also be short, decide to lead an enjoyable, hedonistic lifestyle. When they then die, as expected, earlier than other people, the reduced longevity may be blamed on their external rather than internal risk factors.

Another important susceptibility factor is the human psyche. Many doctors and patients can tell you that people who develop the heart attacks called myocardial infarctions are often tense, driven, with considerable repressed anger and hostility. If such patients also tend to smoke and to eat high fat diets, the heart attacks will be attributed to the external rather than the internal risk factors. Has this psychic feature been checked? No, not really. Instead of using well-constructed psychometric rating methods to identify anger, hostility, and tension, epidemiologists have gotten controversial results by using what may be the world's clumsiest and most oversimplified classification of the complexity of the human psyche. According to the customary epidemiologic rating scale, which is also difficult to reproduce, every human psyche is either a Type A or a Type B. There are many kinds of races, ethnic groups, and even serum lipoproteins in human biology, but in epidemiologic research for risk factors there have been only two types of human psyches. The quality of the associated science resembles what would happen if we divided all chemical exposures into being organic or inorganic.

Another neglected source of susceptibility bias is a factor that my colleagues and I have called protopathic (or "early disease") bias (Horwitz and Feinstein, 1980). It arises when exposure (or nonexposure) is affected by a disease that has begun to produce clinical symptom, but has not yet been recognized. For example, a middle-aged man who has developed the exertional chest pain of angina pectoris, but who has not told anyone about it, may deliberately avoid jogging or other vigorous forms of physical exertion. Later on, when he develops a myocardial infarction, it will be blamed on his slothful lifestyle. The early-disease protopathic problem is seldom recognized, because epidemiologists almost never ask about the baseline state features that can make people choose or avoid certain exposures.

These three types of susceptibility bias produce a confounding that cannot be recognized or adjusted with multivariable analysis, because the necessary data are not acquired and are therefore not available to be analyzed.

Detection bias

The detection bias form of confounding arises when the outcome event is sought and identified with different vigor, methods, or criteria in the exposed and nonexposed groups. In clinical trials of therapy, particularly when a change of symptoms is the outcome event, detection bias is avoided not by randomization, but by double-blind procedures in which neither the patient nor the doctor knows which treatment is being given. The problem arises in a different way in epidemiologic studies of risk factors, where the outcome event is development of a particular disease.

A fundamental difficulty here is that many chronic disease epidemiologists do not seem to know or understand chronic disease. They do not realize that many instances of cancer, coronary disease, and various forms of arteriosclerosis can exist in a clinically "silent" form, being first discerned at a postmortem necropsy done after the patient has died of some other cause. A 90-year-old man, shot by a jealous lover, may show coronary arteries so occluded that one wonders how he was able to walk, let alone engage in the activity that led to his demise. The necropsy may also show that he had a cancer in the lung or in the colon that had previously been asymptomatic and unrecognized.

With so many silent cases of disease available for identification during life, all that is needed to produce detection bias is an exposure that is associated with increased diagnostic searches. Furthermore, all that is needed to raise the occurrence rates of any disease is an improved diagnostic method or wider dissemination and usage of an existing method (Feinstein and Esdaile, 1987).

For example, during the past decade, the increased occurrence rates of brain tumor, breast cancer, and pancreatic cancer have evoked many fears of cancer epidemics and have led to suspicions about risk factors such as electric power lines, microwave ovens, and cellular telephones. Do these rising rates represent real increases in those diseases, or are they due to increased diagnosis during life, with the use of improved technologic methods, such as CAT scans of the head, mammography, and abdominal ultrasound? Knowledgeable clinicians would promptly answer that the rises in occurrence are due to improved diagnosis, but many chronic disease epidemiologists seem to be unaware of this possibility. One of my heretical colleagues has said that many epidemiologists believe disease is something that occurs on a death certificate.

If you ask me to get an industry into trouble, I can promptly tell you how to do so: Set up a mammography screening program. It will identify many breast cancers that were formerly undetected. The high rate of breast cancer in that industry, however, will not be compared against the rate found in some other industry that also has a mammography screening program. Instead, with the customary epidemiologic neglect of detection bias, the rate will be compared against the rate of breast cancer in the general public, for which mammography screening is not yet ubiquitous. The higher breast cancer rate in the industry will then be attributed not to mammography, but to the employees' exposure to whatever product is made by that industry: widgets, chicken soup, dioxin, antibiotics, etc. In mere general studies, various cancers and other diseases become associated with working in or living near industrial sites, and no attention is given to the fact that people in these locations may also be more likely to receive the technologic testing that identifies the disease.

A profound neglect of detection bias is not only one of the major scientific deficiencies of current epidemiologic research, but is also becoming almost a scandal. One study after another is done, often with contradictory results, about alcohol, food, smoking, estrogens, or power lines as risk factors for breast cancer (and other cancers), and none of the studies give adequate attention to suitable methods that could remove the confounding of detection bias.

An even greater scandal, which I do not have time to go into, is the reliance on death certificate data for calculating incidence rates of disease (Gittlesohn and Royston, 1982). A death certificate is merely a civilized passport to burial. The only trustworthy information on a death certificate is the fact and date of death, and the age and sex of the deceased. For more than 50 years, every time someone has studied the causes of death listed on death certificates, the conclusion has been that the information is grossly inaccurate and unreliable, and that a wholly new system is needed for scientifically trustworthy data (Feinstein and Esdaile, 1987; Gittlesohn and Royston, 1982). Yet nothing has been done. In the midst of the magnificent scientific advances of molecular biology and medical technology in the 20th century, the egregiously defective information on death certificates continues to be used for determining incidence rates of disease. The imageries are now augmented with computer-generated maps of the incidence of cancer in different regions.

Transfer bias

After the exposures and outcomes have occurred, the events must be counted in all the pertinent people. In a randomized trial, or in an observational cohort study that follows people forward in time from their exposure (or nonexposure), the group of pertinent people is known and counted at the beginning of the study. If all of them are not suitably accounted for afterwards, the results can be biased when effects related to the exposure (or nonexposure) make people drop out or become lost to follow-up in disproportionate numbers in the two groups.

To avoid these transfer problems, a suitable scientific accounting is usually obtained with life-table analysis, or, in randomized trials, with a so-called "intention to treat analyses". In case-control studies, however, a cohort of exposed and nonexposed persons is not assembled. Not being themselves "exposed" to identifying a baseline state, the investigators often make no provision for what may have transpired, and which persons may have been lost, between the baseline state and the group who are assembled as cases and controls, at the end of the causal pathway, after everything has already happened.

Furthermore, in choosing the cases and controls, investigators can create biases above and beyond what already exists. The research may establish peculiar eligibility criteria that pertain for cases but not controls, or vice versa, so that a form of exclusion bias is almost guaranteed (Horwitz and Feinstein, 1985). Perhaps the most glaring example of the production of transfer bias, however, was committed by one of the most prominent leaders of epidemiologic research. Suppose a pharmaceutical company did a study, analyzed the results, did not like them, and decided to discard members of the control group so that the subsequent results were much more favorable to the research hypothesis. The subsequent scandal would perhaps be front-page news, receiving citation by media anchor-persons and perhaps even getting attention from national science commentators, such as Oprah Winfrey and Geraldo Rivera.

The strategy of changing the control group *after* the data was analyzed was not done by a pharmaceutical company, however, it was done by one of the world's best known epidemiologists, in a famous (or infamous) case-control study that accused reserpine (a then popular blood pressure medication) of causing breast cancer (Armstrong et al., 1974). The authors of the paper did not hide what they had done:

they said so in their published account of methods. Since the prominent epidemiologist has helped set the so-called standards for peer review, however, the paper was accepted and published in one of the world's leading medical journals. The accusation later turned out to be wrong, and reserpine was eventually exonerated, but as far as I know the offending paper has never been retracted.

Exposure bias

I have saved exposure bias, as a fourth source of confounding, for emphasis now, because it is specifically cited in the title assigned for this talk. In most epidemiologic studies, and in all case-control studies, the ascertainment of exposure is a retrospective process, conducted after the events have actually occurred. The ascertainment involves either a search through archival records, or a direct interview with the research subjects, or both. The ascertainment process surely warrants special procedures to ensure objectivity, such as the double-blinding used to ascertain the outcome events in a clinical trial. For example, when my colleagues and I do case-control studies, we establish special methods of recruiting and interviewing subjects to keep the interviewers from knowing who is a case and who is a control, and even to keep the interviewed subjects themselves from knowing whether they are cases or controls. We also set up a series of "decoy hypotheses" so that the interviewers will not know the particular exposure in which we are most interested (Feinstein, 1985).

In most epidemiologic studies, however, no such efforts are made. In fact, one prominent leader in epidemiology has reportedly said that such efforts, which are now used routinely by myself and colleagues, are impossible. Consequently, in most studies, the interviewers usually know who a case is and who a control is; and they also know what hypothesis the investigator is trying to prove. The approach creates almost unlimited opportunities for interviewer bias by the researcher, and for recall bias by the subject. If you tell me what exposure you are looking for, and tell me the state of the person I am interviewing, I should be able to elicit a positive history in people whom you want to have it, and a negative history in people who should not. Yet almost no precautions are taken to avoid this type of bias in ascertaining exposure. Furthermore, since the bias is incorporated directly into the raw data, its existence is impossible to prove afterward.

When the possibility of ascertainment bias is raised, many epidemiologists will retort, "You haven't proved it". This is a strange reply in scientific research, where the investigator's job is to take suitable precautions. For example, if a randomized trial is done without the precautions of pertinent double-blinding, the results will usually be rejected summarily, without anyone having to prove anything about bias. If a surgeon tries to enter an operating room with dirty hands, he (or she) will usually be promptly ejected, without anyone having to demonstrate any bacteria on the hands. In epidemiologic chronic disease research, however, it is perfectly acceptable for the investigators to take no precautions against exposure bias, and then, if you complain, to demand you prove that bias occurred.

I shall mention, only in passing, a separate problem in biased exposure. In many studies, the investigators do not identify, in advance, what they mean by *exposure*. Instead, they acquire the data, examine the results, and then demarcate exposure retrospectively in a way that is most favorable for whatever hypothesis they want to prove.

Reasons for problems

At this point, you are probably wondering whether things are really as bad as I have stated. I regret to tell you that yes, they are. If you then ask why things have gotten and remained this way, I can offer several sets of explanations.

The first is that chronic disease epidemiology is still a relatively young and developing field, in which scientific methods are particularly difficult to use, because intact human beings cannot be studied with the same ease as inanimate substances, caged animals, or molecules. Because all domains of science develop at their own pace, there is absolutely no reason why this young field should be as methodologically well-developed, sophisticated, and mature today as chemistry or physics. Even the marvels of molecular biology are only about 40 years old.

If scientific methodologic errors still occur in chronic disease epidemiology, there is nothing shameful about them. As the field advances, they will be improved. If the idea of shame is to be raised, however, we can surely be embarrassed by the folly of believing that chronic disease epidemiology is well advanced scientifically, and then giving serious credibility to results that would be instantly dismissed if presented in many other branches of science (Feinstein, 1988).

A second major reason for problems, is the difficulty of reproducing the research. If someone claims to have achieved cold fusion in a physics laboratory, physicists all over the world can go into their own laboratories and try to repeat the work. In epidemiology, however, you can never get exactly the same group of people to be examined in exactly the same place, in exactly the same way, and for exactly the same duration. For this reason, the problem of suitable methodology is particularly important. Because the *material* itself cannot be reproduced, the methods have to be particularly effective and persuasive. In this respect, however, many leaders of the field have been particularly delinquent. They have done relatively little to improve the shoddy methods I have described; they have sometimes been responsible for creating those methods; and they often reinforce the shoddiness in their work as peer reviewers for grant requests and journal manuscripts.

The third major problem, which leads to tolerance of the methodologic shoddiness, is a frequent focus on mathematical rather than scientific models for scientific research. Many chronic disease epidemiologists, for example, will argue that case-control studies and other epidemiologic research structures are special kinds of scientific research that should be judged with their own principles and standards, not with the same criteria used in other branches of science. Since an observational epidemiologic study is not a randomized trial, and since the chronic-disease investigators do not regard the studies as a substitute for a randomized trial, the investigators will state that the work does not require and should not be judged by any of the other scientific standards that are applied in randomized trials. In the views of these investigators, case-control and other epidemiologic studies can be approached with the rules of statistical inference, but no rules have been established for scientific inference.

A fourth major problem, which also encourages the tolerance of shoddy methods, is the role of social and political advocacy in public health. Clinical practitioners are often reproached for their God-like attitudes in believing they know what's good for individual patients. Public-health epidemiologists, however, may sometimes have an even larger amount of self-deification in believing they know what's good for the world. Once they believe that something is evil — whether it be food, sloth, or fun — anything that can help to get rid of that evil is acceptable research, regardless of the scientific quality of the methods. Although scientific investigation usually insists that the end is justified only if the means are justified, in many forms of epidemiologic research, the end justifies the means.

The advocacy has now become particularly troublesome, because it has begun to be used by governmental agencies, armed with regulatory authority, to pervert epidemiology into political science. In the former Soviet Union, biological science has not yet recovered from the intellectual degeneration it suffered when the scientific fantasies of Lysenko, which were compatible with Soviet political policy, became adopted as scientific policy. Instead of developing improved methods, epidemiological science in the United States, will probably go through a similar degeneration if it is transmogrified into an analogous form of Lysenkoism, used to advance the advocacy and political goals of governmental agencies. A recent oasis in the increasingly desolate scientific desert of certain public-health agencies was the confession by one former agency director that he was wrong when he ordered an entire town in Missouri evacuated about a decade ago because of a risk factor threat that turned out not to be a threat. A few more confessions of that type might be particularly salubrious for science in the world of risk-factor opportunism and public health advocacy.

The last problem I shall cite is that if schools of medicine can (quite properly) be indicted for their failure to teach generalism and humanism, schools of public health — which have spawned so many chronic disease epidemiologists — can be indicted for their failure to teach disease or science or a scientific attitude of searching for errors. The students seldom have any laboratory courses to give direct experience in doing experiments; there are almost no courses in pathology, physiology, or diagnosis to teach about disease; there is no exposure to autopsies that can teach about latent disease and diagnostic error; and in fact, there is no established tradition of searching for error in teaching rounds or other special conferences. Several years ago, when Vandenbroucke and Pardoel (1989) published an intellectual "autopsy" to analyze the error in which amyl nitrite poppers were initially regarded as the cause of AIDS, I realized it was the first such paper I had seen in the epidemiologic literature.

Until improvements begin to appear routinely in the scientific quality of the work,

38

we shall continue to be stuck with epidemiologic claims about risk factors and to confront the problems of deciding when the claims warrant credibility. I do not think routine methodologic improvements will come quickly, because I doubt that the older generation of leaders in chronic disease epidemiology will try to institute reforms in the defective methods that they have created, disseminated, built into the peer review process, coerced into grant approvals, and used as foundations and stepping stones for their careers and elevated status. There is always hope, of course, for the younger generation, and particularly for the generation that follows them. Furthermore, if things become too decadent in our own country or in other English-speaking countries, there is always hope for other parts of the world.

Eventually truth and science will triumph. Until that splendid time arrives, however, we shall have to be careful to remember that statistical associations, even when embellished or adumbrated by multivariable analytic miracles, are not necessarily scientific evidence.

References

Armstrong B, Stevens N and Doll R. Retrospective study of the association between use of rauwolfia derivatives and breast cancer in English women. Lancet 1974;2:672–675.

Cornfield J. Statistical relationships and proof in medicine. Am Stat 1954;8:19–21.

Feinstein AR. Clinical Epidemiology. The Architecture of Clinical Research. Philadelphia: W.B. Saunders Co. 1985.

Feinstein AR. Scientific standards in epidemiologic studies of the menace of daily life. Science 1988;242:1257–1263.

Feinstein AR. Epidemiologic analyses of causation: the unlearned scientific lessons of randomized trials. J Clin Edidemiol 1989;42:481–489.

Feinstein AR and Esdaile JM. Incidence, prevalence, and evidence. Scientific problems in epidemiologic statistics for the occurrence of cancer. Am J Med 1987;82:113–123.

Gittlesohn A and Royston PN. Annotated bibliography of cause-of-death validation studies 1958–80. Washington DC: U.S. Government Printing Office, 1982. (Vital and Health Statistics. Series 2, No. 89) (DHHS Publication No. [PHS] 82–1363).

Greenland S and Morganstern H. Classification schemes for epidemiologic research designs. J Clin Epidemiol 1988;42:715–716.

Horwitz RI and Feinstein AR. The problem of "protopathic bias" in case-control studies. Am J Med 1980;68:255–258.

Horwitz RI and Feinstein AR. Exclusion bias and the false relationship or reserpine and breast cancer. Arch Int Med 1985;145:1873–1875.

Miettinen OS. Striving to deconfound the fundamentals of epidemiologic study design. J Clin Epidemiol 1988;41:709–713.

Rothman KJ. Modern Epidemiology. Boston: Little, Brown and Co., 1986.

Vandenbroucke JP and Pardoel VPAM. An autopsy of epidemiologic methods: the case of "poppers" in the early epidemic of the acquired immunodeficiency syndrome (AIDS). Am J Epidemiol 1989;129:455–457.

©1995 Elsevier Science B.V. All rights reserved.
The Role of Epidemiology in Regulatory Risk Assessment
J.D. Graham, editor.

Epidemiology: bias bias everywhere? And not one drop of science?

Allan H. Smith

Department of Biomedical and Environmental Health Sciences, University of California, Berkeley, California, USA

Key words: bias, confounding, consistency, dose-response, epidemiology, extrapolation, risk assessment, selection.

I have read with considerable interest the article by Dr Feinstein. With elegant language and, at times, fiery passion, he appears to demolish the edifice called epidemiology. In this discussion I wish to focus on the following topics:
1. What is epidemiology?
2. Why is it that epidemiologists have achieved the reputation of internal dissention: never being able to agree among themselves?
3. Are all epidemiological studies biased?
4. The degree of bias in epidemiological studies?
5. The bias in extrapolating human risks from rodents?
6. Future directions in the use of epidemiology in risk assessment.

What is epidemiology?

Epidemiology is sometimes vaguely defined in jargon that confuses it with statistical exercises. For example, "epidemiology is the study of disease occurrence in human populations" or "epidemiology is the study of the distribution and determinants of disease in human populations". Such definitions avoid the obvious. Since epidemiology involves studying groups of people, and since it is only by studying groups of people (both patients with disease and those not so afflicted) that one can determine the cause of diseases in humans, any appropriate definition should include the word "cause". I was therefore pleased to note that Dr Feinstein opened his paper by referring to the epidemiological appraisal as a cause-effect analysis. He might not agree though with my favorite definition of epidemiology:

> Epidemiology is the science which studies the causes of disease in human populations and how to prevent them.

Address for correspondence: Allan H. Smith, Department of Biomedical and Environmental Health Sciences, University of California-B, Berkeley, CA 94720, USA. Tel.: +1-510-843-1763. Fax: +1-510-843-5539.

In support of this definition, I would again note that no cause of disease in humans can be confirmed without a human population study. The latest disease-related discoveries of molecular biology have to be confirmed and elucidated by epidemiological studies. I would also note that, while it is true that epidemiologists collect population data on disease rates and trends, the ultimate purpose for doing so usually relates to ascertaining causes of disease and preventing them. In this regard, it is my belief that we should keep a clear distinction between epidemiology addressing disease causation and various uses of health statistics, such as in health services research where disease incidence trends might be collected for health services planning.

Why do I commence by defining epidemiology in discussing Dr Feinstein's paper? It is because when defined in this way, it is apparent that for all the flaws in epidemiological studies, we have no choice but to use epidemiology in identifying disease causation in humans. We may gradually improve the scientific quality of epidemiological studies as Dr Feinstein wishes, but we have to use what we have got now in human risk assessment. Looked at in this way, I suggest we should focus more on what is right about epidemiology today, than what is wrong about it. Use of the well established key criteria for causal inference: consistency, strength of association, dose-response, and time relationships, has led to many important conclusions about disease causation which have stood the test of time.

Why is it that epidemiologists have achieved the reputation of internal dissension: never being able to agree among themselves?

I think a major epidemiological bias we confront, and one not raised by Dr Feinstein, is that epidemiologists are notorious for criticizing each other's work and never agreeing on anything. I have often wondered why this is. Other scientists disagree too, but seem to reach consensus more rapidly. They look on and say, if epidemiologists can never agree amongst themselves, how can we give credence to epidemiology? Dr Feinstein discusses some of the reasons for this. He notes for example, that it is more difficult to reproduce epidemiological research, than laboratory research. However, I believe there is another reason which relates to the fact that epidemiology is often producing information on which critical policy and regulatory decisions are made. These decisions affect many vested interests who move to defend their turf by hiring epidemiologists to criticize the work of other epidemiologists. The appearance to the outsider is that epidemiologists can never agree. My own experience is that epidemiologists often reach consensus fairly readily until the hired gun epidemiologist comes into the picture.

Are all epidemiological studies biased?

The simple answer to this question is yes. Observational studies inevitably have potential biases not present in well controlled experiments. In graduate classes at Berkeley, I regularly give a lecture titled "Epidemiology is always biased; and ever so interesting because of it". In that lecture, I hold a recent issue of an epidemiology journal upside down, and randomly open it at a page. I then say this study is full of biases. The three major types of bias are all present; selection bias, information bias and confounding. Selection bias is present because the comparison populations differ from the study population with regard to education, socioeconomic status and other variables. If it is a case-control study, there are problems with the selection of the control group. With regard to information bias, there is potential bias due to misclassification of diagnoses and the exposure data are crude and of dubious validity. With regard to confounding, several potential confounding factors have been omitted from the study, and there is still residual confounding from those included due to inaccuracy and imprecision in the measurement of confounding factors. There are also at least ten other biases in the study. I then turn the journal up the right way. Nine times out of ten, everything I have said is correct.

The degree of bias in epidemiological studies

In the same lecture referred to above, I then go on to point out that in most epidemiological studies only one or two potential biases are really a matter of concern. The others produce little bias, or perhaps produce a small bias towards finding no effect. Furthermore, it is often possible to put limits on the main potential biases, and one can usually identify the most likely direction of the bias. An example of this is confounding. It is very rare for confounding to result in a relative risk greater than 1.5, and almost never greater than 2, unless the study has been very poorly designed.

The bias in extrapolating human risks from rodents

Potential biases in epidemiological studies used for risk assessment need to be contrasted with the potential bias in extrapolating risks from experiments on rodents. It is sometimes made to appear that when there is both rodent and human data, the risk estimates are reasonably close. Such comparisons are quite spurious. There are a variety of assumptions which go into risk assessment from both types of data, and these assumptions are usually juggled to bring the risk estimates closer. For example, whether or not to make metabolic rate corrections in extrapolating from rodents is usually decided after seeing how the epidemiological and rodent risk estimates compare.

Some idea of the potential uncertainties in estimating risks from rodents can be gained by examining extrapolations from mice to rats and vice versa. In reviewing studies in mice and rats, it has been noted that in only 74% of the cases are chemicals tested for carcinogenicity active in both species (Haseman and Lockhard,

1993). Furthermore, in less than 36% is there site specific agreement. In other words, if one used mice to predict whether or not a chemical would cause a specific cancer in rats (or vice versa), one would be wrong in the majority of cases. The picture is even worse for lung cancer since there is no correlation between the two species. One might just as well roll dice rather than use mice to predict whether or not a chemical will cause rats to get lung cancer. And this applies just to predicting whether or not the substance will cause cancer, let alone predicting risk.

In the light of the order of magnitude uncertainties in predicting cancer risks from rodents, it is my view that epidemiological data should be given priority in predicting human cancer risks. For example, uncertainties in exposure of the order of 2 (i.e., exposure might be 2 times higher or 2 times lower than estimated) are trivial in comparison to the uncertainties in extrapolating risks from rodents to humans.

Future directions in the use of epidemiology in risk assessment

The use of epidemiological data for risk assessment is likely to increase in the future, but the problems will not go away. As Dr Feinstein points out, exposure data are critical, and we all hope to see improvements in this area, ideally with increased use of biological markers of exposure. However, since we will increasingly be using epidemiological studies to identify lower and lower environmental risks, such as from air pollution and relatively low exposure to chemicals, improvements in study design are not likely to make the use of epidemiological data less difficult and controversial. The uncertainties may in fact increase. Methods for estimating risks from epidemiological studies in the face of uncertainty warrant careful attention. However, the goal of disease prevention means that, instead of tearing epidemiological studies apart, we need to examine them systematically for use in risk assessment knowing that there are no better alternative approaches.

Reference

Haseman JK and Lockhart A-M. Correlations between chemically related site-specific carcinogenic effects in long-term studies in rats and mice. Environ Health Perspect 1993;101(1):50–54.

©1995 Elsevier Science B.V. All rights reserved.
The Role of Epidemiology in Regulatory Risk Assessment
J.D. Graham, editor.

An evaluation of biases introduced by confounding and imperfect retrospective and prospective exposure assessments

Christine M. Friedenreich

Department of Community Health Sciences, The University of Calgary, Calgary, Alberta, Canada

Key words: bias, confounding, design, epidemiology, exposure, prospective, retrospective, risk.

Introduction

Dr Feinstein (1995) has succinctly outlined a number of the methodologic concerns with epidemiologic studies that need to be considered when the results of these studies are used in regulatory risk assessment. These concerns center on the inability of observational epidemiologic studies to control for all extraneous factors, besides those under investigation, as is undertaken in a randomized controlled trial. Since epidemiologists are often restricted to observing human populations and examining cause-effect relations through either retrospective or prospective measurements of exposure, they do not have the same level of "control" over the experiment as would a basic scientist or a clinician undertaking a randomized trial. Rather, epidemiologists have developed methods, that are still rapidly evolving, to capture the exposure experience of a population and to relate this to their disease occurrence. They examine the strength, consistency, specificity, dose-response, temporality, and biologic plausibility of these putative associations and consider the influence of biases on the direction of the effects being measured. Dr Feinstein has raised numerous concerns regarding the scientific standards in observational epidemiologic studies and, in particular, whether the results of these studies are inherently biased, confounded and not to be trusted. These concerns, regarding biases and confounding, will be addressed and suggestions provided for how epidemiologic methods may be studied and improved and how epidemiologic study results may be used in regulatory risk assessment.

Types of bias in epidemiologic studies

Dr Feinstein describes biases that may arise in identifying the diseased population

---

Address for correspondence: Christine M. Friedenreich PhD, Department of Community Health Sciences, The University of Calgary, 3330 Hospital Drive NW, Calgary, Alberta, Canada T2N 4N1. Tel.: +1-403-220-8242 (5110). Fax: +1-403-283-4740.

(i.e., susceptibility bias, detection bias, transfer bias) and in measuring the exposures (i.e., interviewer bias, recall bias). These biases are a few of the numerous biases previously defined (Sackett, 1979; Last, 1988). For this presentation, biases will be categorized into three main types: biases in the sampling of the outcome, biases in the exposure measurement, and confounding. Each major group of biases will be described and suggestions for minimizing the effect of these biases in epidemiologic research presented.

Biases in outcome sampling

Biases in outcome sampling arise when the subjects selected for the study are not representative of the base population from which they are chosen. This situation may occur when study subjects either select themselves for the study by volunteering to participate (i.e., self-selection bias), when subjects are selected from a cohort that is systematically different from the base population (e.g., healthy workers), when subjects are selected because of a diagnostic procedure that identifies them that is not available to the entire population (i.e., diagnostic bias), or when subjects who agree to participate are systematically different from those who do not respond (i.e., nonrespondent bias). As Dr Feinstein has mentioned, bias in outcome sampling is also possible if persons who are more susceptible to develop the disease are chosen preferentially over those who do not share this susceptibility (susceptibility bias) or when the outcome event is sought more vigorously among the exposed population (detection bias).

Since epidemiologic studies always require that the base population be sampled, strategies are needed to ensure that the study sample is representative of that base population. This conference is focused on regulatory risk assessment, and an example of a key area of risk assessment is identifying potential carcinogens, quantifying the risk associated with these carcinogens, and preventing potential future exposures. Studies of cancer risks are facilitated by the use of population-based cancer registries where a complete record of all occurrences of clinical cancer can be readily obtained. Similar reporting of incident cases exists for certain infectious diseases, congenital anomalies, childhood injuries, and some, but not all, chronic diseases (e.g., diabetes mellitus, some forms of cardiovascular and cerebrovascular disease, renal disease, Alzheimer's disease). These registries will, however, not include undetected cases of disease. In order to include cases that are subclinical, registries of early detection activities (e.g., screening programs for cancer) are needed. As Dr Feinstein has noted, death certificates are not a valid method for estimating disease incidence, in fact, they actually record prevalent disease. Better methods, such as mandatory registration of chronic diseases and diagnostic activities, are clearly needed and are, indeed, being used more frequently. Of importance to note are the increasing ethical and legal issues that are being raised with the use of registries. Scientists must be supportive of this type of population registration since epidemiologic studies will become even more difficult and biased without this means of disease estimation.

Recognizing the possibility of bias in a particular study design and population sampling method is the first step, when designing a study, towards avoiding this bias. As Dr Feinstein and others have clearly described, several of the biases in outcome sampling can be avoided simply by choosing a population sampling strategy that does not involve a highly selected population that is unrepresentative of the base population. This awareness can mitigate the possibility of numerous biases enumerated here. Attaining high response rates in epidemiologic studies also minimizes the problem of nonresponse bias. Mitigating the effect of susceptibility bias presents a greater challenge for epidemiologists. In order to assess the baseline state of an individual *before* an exposure to a putative risk factor occurs, a prospective, long-term follow-up study may be necessary. These studies, however, are not always viable or cost-efficient. In retrospective studies, this bias may be minimized by obtaining information from the study subject on their characteristics of importance provided these can be readily recalled. Advances in genetic and molecular epidemiology may soon permit assessments to be made of a study subject's genetic predisposition for disease. These assessments could, potentially, be free of any reporting bias and would provide the type of information on the baseline state that Dr Feinstein is suggesting needs to be considered.

An additional note of caution regarding biases in outcome sampling is the need for valid comparison groups. Bias in the selection of controls is an important and widely recognized weakness of retrospective studies. An investigator must ensure that both cases and controls are representative of the base population and that the controls, had they become cases, would have been included in the study population (Rothman, 1986).

Biases in exposure measurement

Biases in exposure measurement arise if systematic errors are made when obtaining (i.e., interviewer bias) or when reporting information on exposure (i.e., recall or reporting bias). Interviewer bias can occur when interviewers are aware of the study hypotheses and use different interviewing strategies for the diseased and nondiseased populations. Likewise, recall bias may occur if study subjects are aware of the hypothesis under investigation and systematically over or underestimate their exposure levels. These biases are of greatest concern in retrospective studies that rely on interview-administered reports of past exposures. Both prospective and retrospective studies may be subject to misclassification of exposures; however, this is a random rather than a systematic type of error that is considered nondifferential (i.e., not related to the outcome status) and that results in an underestimation of the risk (Barron, 1977; Copeland et al., 1977; Raphael, 1987; Coughlin, 1990). Since this paper is focusing on systematic errors that result in overestimations of risk (i.e., away from the null value), exposure misclassification will not be discussed further.

As Dr Feinstein has suggested, interviewer bias may be removed or at least minimized by "blinding" the interviewers to the case and control status of the subjects and the hypotheses under investigation. Unfortunately for some diseases it is not possible to hide the case or control status of the study subject from the interviewer. In these situations, careful interviewer training including the need for impartiality in the interviews must be particularly emphasized. Regular monitoring of interviews should also be a routine procedure in any study using interviewers. With respect to "blinding" the study subjects, usually the particular disease-exposure relation being studied, can be hidden, however, ethics committees sometimes demand that subjects know what the study hypotheses are since they consider protecting the rights of the individual more important than the need to mitigate a respondent bias.

Recall bias is widely considered a major methodologic concern in epidemiologic studies. However, relatively few studies have specifically been designed to examine the presence of recall bias and the results have been inconsistent (Drews et al., 1990; Feldman et al., 1989; Floderus, 1990; Friedenreich 1991; Klemetti and Saxén, 1967; Mackenzie and Lippman, 1989; Schull and Cobb, 1969; Stolly et al., 1978; Tilly et al., 1985; UK National Case-control Study Group, 1989; Weinstock et al., 1991; Werler et al., 1989; Giovannucci et al., 1993). Recall bias may be comprised of a so-called social desirability bias. This bias probably has two components. On the one hand, study subjects may underestimate their exposures to "bad" habits such as smoking, alcohol drinking, and eating of high fat foods and, on the other hand, overestimate exposures to "good" habits such as exercise. Furthermore, they may also overestimate their exposures to environmental or external factors (e.g., chemical exposures) over which they have no control and that they can "blame" for their disease. Hence, recall bias is a complex bias that clearly needs to be studied more carefully but that may not necessarily be inevitable in retrospective studies.

Factors that influence recall require more attention in epidemiologic studies. Recent research examining the processes underlying recall bias has shown that a respondent's mood or state of mind may influence recall (Raphael and Cloitre, 1994). Indeed, it was shown that mood rather than case status per se may have a biasing effect.

When designing studies, epidemiologists should also consider the thought processes that a respondent undergoes when recalling past exposures (Friedenreich, 1994). Cognitive psychologists and survey researchers have identified the four cognitive processes used when answering a question (Tourangeau, 1984). These processes are: question comprehension, information retrieval, estimation/judgement, and response formulation. For each process, they have developed and tested methods to improve the subject's ability to recall retrospective exposures. Examples of methods used to improve reporting and recall are laboratory and field pretesting of questionnaires, and cognitive interviewing, which includes strategies such as a personal time line, memory probes, paraphrasing, and emphasizing the need for honest responses (Bercini, 1992; Means et al., 1991; Jobe and Mingay, 1989).

Another potential method for reducing biases in exposure measurement is the use of biologic markers of exposure (Hulka et al., 1990). Biologic markers offer the possibility of obtaining valid exposure information free from reporting errors or bias. Unfortunately, few time-integrated, long-term markers of exposure currently exist.

However, this is a rapidly evolving field that holds promise for studies of environmental and occupational exposures.

Avoiding or, at least, mitigating biases in exposure assessment is an underlying tenet for the proper conduct of epidemiologic studies. Nonetheless, instances arise when biases may occur. The effect of biases resulting from errors in exposure assessment is being quantified and their influence on the magnitude and direction of risk estimates is being assessed (Marshall et al., 1981; Walker and Blettner, 1985; Walter and Irwig, 1988; Flegal et al., 1991; Reade-Christopher and Kupper, 1991; Walker and Lanes, 1991; Brenner and Blettner, 1993; Brenner et al., 1993). Furthermore, methods that reduce or remove the influence of these biases are being designed and applied in epidemiologic studies (Savitz and Baron, 1989; Rosner et al., 1990; Liu and Liang, 1991; Phillips and Davey Smith, 1993; Kaaks, 1994).

For epidemiologic study results to be applicable to regulatory risk assessment, appropriate data on exposures must be collected. To begin, relatively few exposures for which regulation may be required have been examined in epidemiologic studies. Secondly, lifetime cumulative exposures (i.e., dose) have often been inadequately measured, if at all (Matanoski, 1988). Thirdly, the latency period between the exposure(s) and disease outcome(s) is not consistently considered in the analyses (Matanoski, 1988). Finally, to overcome these problems in exposure measurement, closer collaboration between epidemiologists and laboratory scientists is needed to ensure that the data needed by risk assessors are properly collected and analyzed.

Confounding

As Dr Feinstein has clearly pointed out in his paper, confounding is a particular concern in observational epidemiologic studies, although it also exists in experimental research. When considering exposure-outcome relations in epidemiologic studies, the effects of other factors may influence the relation being studied. In order to be a confounder, a factor must be related to both the exposure and to the outcome being studied *and* it must be predictive of the outcome independent of the exposure (Rothman, 1986). A factor that is a step in the causal pathway between exposure and disease is not a confounder. It has also been demonstrated that other factors, not on the causal pathway but that change the effect of an exposure, should not be considered as confounders or effect modifiers since adjusting for these factors may actually severely bias risk estimates (Weinberg, 1993).

When assessing the validity of epidemiologic study results, investigators and users of the results must clearly understand the underlying biologic model in order to assess whether the exposure-disease relation is true or whether it could be explained by uncontrolled confounding. In experimental studies, the effects of confounding factors are generally considered to be unimportant since they are, supposedly, evenly distributed between the two groups being compared. In observational studies, confounding factors may invalidate the results if they are not properly considered in the study design and analysis. Hence, in prospective studies, investigators must know *a priori* which outcome(s) they are measuring in their study population and which factors may confound the exposure-outcome relation(s) being studied. Likewise, in retrospective studies, a full examination of potential confounding factors is necessary. The challenge, however, is being able to differentiate factors that are on the causal pathway from those that are true confounders. More research effort needs to be placed on examining factors that are linked and determining what is their role in the cause-effect relation. Although inconsistencies in epidemiologic study results may occur because of the different study samples and measurement methods used, they may also result from the widely different confounding factors controlled for in the analysis. Thus, as Dr Feinstein has suggested, there is a need for a common understanding of the biology behind a specific cause-effect relation being studied in order that the confounding factors of importance be adequately measured and controlled for in the analysis.

Application of epidemiologic research to regulatory risk assessment

Dr Feinstein has argued that political advocacy in public health research should be avoided and has clearly expressed his concerns that epidemiology may suffer if political considerations are permitted to influence epidemiologic research or the interpretation of epidemiologic study results. The onus on epidemiologists is to conduct methodologically sound, valid research that makes significant contributions to knowledge and that withstands intense scrutiny. A further need exists for epidemiologists to interpret their study results to nonepidemiologists and explain the likelihood that the cause-effect relation is real and not attributable to biases in the sample, design, exposure measurement, or analysis. Epidemiologists are often pressured to publicize strong positive or negative findings and to provide immediate public health recommendations, yet, extreme caution is generally needed in making these recommendations since no single study is definitive. On the other hand, epidemiologists have a duty to make recommendations when evidence for a risk is strong and when negative population health consequences may exist.

Another area of concern with respect to confounding and biases, discussed elsewhere in this conference, is how the results of epidemiologic studies should be pooled and summarized for regulatory purposes. When conducting either a pooled or meta-analysis to summarize the findings of previously conducted studies, consideration must be given to how any biases and confounding may have influenced the results from these studies. In particular, are the risk estimates likely to be over or underestimated because of systematic errors introduced by a biased study sample, study methods or analysis? Should study results be pooled if biases are believed to have influenced the results? Further consideration must also be given to the methods and quality of the studies and whether they should be equally weighted in the overview analyses (Friedenreich, 1993). Efforts are on-going to establish methods and mechanisms for the systematic review of randomized controlled trials (Chalmers, 1993); however, similar methods have not yet been established for the systematic review of observational epidemiologic studies. Conducting a proper review of the literature for regulatory or other purposes is challenging since the reviewer must decide whether the results are valid and precise and whether the study was rigorously conducted. To assist these reviews, epidemiologists should provide a detailed description in their publications of their study materials and methods so that other researchers can assess the potential influence of biases and confounding on the presented results. Furthermore, epidemiologists should be willing to share their data for pooled analyses.

Conclusion

Although numerous problems with epidemiologic studies have been described, an equal number of methods to reduce the influence of these potential biases have been provided. Epidemiologists are examining biases empirically, devising methods for reducing biases in outcome sampling and exposure measurement, and improving epidemiologic analytic methods. To improve the applicability of epidemiologic study results to regulatory risk assessment, closer collaboration between epidemiologists and risk assessors is needed to ensure that the necessary data are collected for each process of risk assessment (i.e., hazard identification, dose-response assessment, exposure assessment and risk characterization). The on-going challenge for epidemiologists is to provide human data for regulatory risk assessment that are unbiased, precise, and relevant.

Acknowledgements

Discussion of a paper delivered by Dr Alvan R. Feinstein at the Federal Focus Conference on the Proper Role of Epidemiology in Regulatory Risk Assessment, Lansdowne, VA, USA, October 13, 1994. While writing this paper, C.M. Friedenreich was supported by a full-time fellowship from the Alberta Heritage Foundation for Medical Research.

References

Barron BA. Effects of misclassification on the estimation of relative risk. Biometrics 1977;33:414–418.
Bercini DH. Pretesting questionnaires in the laboratory: an alternative approach. J Exp Anal Envir Epidemiol 1992;2:241–248.
Brenner H and Blettner M. Misclassification bias arising from random error in exposure measurement: implications for dual measurement strategies. Am J Epidemiol 1993;138:453–460.
Brenner H, Savitz and Gefeller O. The effects of joint misclassification of exposure and disease on epidemiologic measures of association. J Clin Epidemiol 1993;46:1195–1202.
Chalmers I. The Cochrane collaboration: preparing, maintaining and disseminating systematic reviews of the effects of health care. Ann NY Acad Sci 1993;703:156–163.
Copeland KT, Checkoway H, McMichael AJ and Holdbrook RH. Bias due to misclassification in the

estimation of relative risk. Am J Epidemiol 1977;105:488–495.

Coughlin SS. Recall bias in epidemiologic studies. J Clin Epidemiol 1990;43:87–91.

Drews CD, Kraus JF and Greenland S. Recall bias in a case-control study of sudden infant death syndrome. Int J Epidemiol 1990;19:405–411.

Feinstein AR. Biases introduced by confounding and imperfect retrospective and prospective exposure assessments. In Graham JD (ed), The Role of Epidemiology in Regulatory Risk Assessment 1995.

Feldman Y, Koren G, Mattice D, Shear H, Pellegrini E and MacLeod S. Determinants of recall and recall bias in studying drug and chemical exposure in pregnancy. Teratology 1989;40:37–45.

Flegal KM, Keyl PM and Nieto FJ. Differential misclassification arising from nondifferential errors in exposure measurement. Am J Epidemiol 1991;134:1233–1244.

Floderus, B. Recall bias in subjective reports of familial cancer. Epidemiol 1990;1:318–321.

Friedenreich CM. Improving long-term recall in epidemiologic studies. Epidemiol 1994;5:1–4.

Friedenreich CM. Methods for pooled analyses of epidemiologic studies. Epidemiol 1993;4:295–302.

Friedenreich CM, Howe GR and Miller AB. The effect of recall bias on the association of calorie-providing nutrients and breast cancer. Epidemiol 1991;2:424–429.

Giovannucci E, Stampfer MJ, Colditz GA, Manson JE, Rosner BA, Longnecker M, Speizer FE and Willett WC. A comparison of prospective and retrospective assessments of diet in the study of breast cancer. Am J Epidemiol 1993;137:502–511.

Hulka BS, Wilcosky TC and Griffith JD. Biological Markers in Epidemiology. Oxford: Oxford University Press, 1990.

Jobe JB and Mingay DJ. Cognitive research improves questionnaires. Am J Public Health 1989;79:-1053–1055.

Kaaks R. Adjustment for bias due to errors in exposure assessments in multicenter cohort studies on diet and cancer: a calibration approach. Am J Clin Nutr 1994;59:245S–250S.

Klemetti A and Saxén L. Prospective versus retrospective approach in the search for environmental causes of malformations. Am J Publ Health 1967;57:2071–2075.

Last JM. A Dictionary of Epidemiology. Toronto: Oxford University Press, 1988 (pp. 13–16).

Liu XH and Liang K-Y. Adjustment for non-differential misclassification error in the generalized linear model. Stat Med 1991;10:1197–1211.

Mackenzie SG and Lippman A. An investigation of report bias in a case-control study of pregnancy outcome. Am J Epidemiol 1989;129:65–75.

Marshall JR, Priore R, Graham S and Brasure J. On the distortion of risk estimates in multiple exposure level case-control studies. Am J Epidemiol 1981;113:464–473.

Matanoski GM. Issues in the measurement of exposure. In: Gordis L (ed), Epidemiology and Health Risk Assessment. New York: Oxford University Press, 1988 (pp. 107–119).

Means B, Swan GE, Jobe JB and Esposito JL. An alternative approach to obtaining personal history data. In: Beimer PP, Groves RM, Lyberg LE, Mathiowetz NA and Sudman S (eds), Measurement Errors in Surveys. New York: John Wiley and Sons, 1991 (pp. 167–183).

Phillips AN and Davey Smith G. The design of prospective epidemiological studies: more subjects or better measurements? J Clin Epidemiol 1993;10:1203–1211.

Raphael K. Recall bias: a proposal for assessment and control. Int J Epidemiol 1987;16:167–170.

Raphael KG and Cloitre M. Does mood-congruence or causal search govern recall bias? A test of life event recall. J Clin Epidemiol 1994;47:555–564.

Reade-Christopher SJ and Kupper LL. Effects of exposure misclassification on regression analyses of epidemiologic follow-up study data. Biometrics 1991;47:535–548.

Rosner B, Spiegelman D and Willett W. Correction of logistic regression relative risk estimates and confidence intervals for measurement error: the case of multiple covariates measured with error. Am J Epidemiol 1990;132:734–745.

Rothman KJ. Modern Epidemiology. Boston: Little, Brown, Co, 1986.

Sackett DL. Bias in analytic research. J Chron Dis 1979;32:51–63.

Savitz DA and Baron AE. Estimating and correcting for confounder misclassification. Am J Epidemiol 1989;129:1062–1071.

Schull WJ and Cobb S. The intrafamilial transmission of rheumatoid arthritis — III. The lack of support for a genetic hypothesis. J Chron Dis 1969;22:217—222.

Stolley PD, Tonascia JA, Sartwell PE, Tockman NS, Toscia S, Rutledge A and Schinnar R. Agreement rates between oral contraceptive users and prescribers in relation to drug use histories. Am J Epidemiol 1978;107:226—235.

Tilley BC, Barnes AB, Bertgstralh E, Labarthe D, Noller KL, Colton T and Adam E. A comparison of pregnancy history recall and medical records. Am J Epidemiol 1985;121:269—281.

Tourangeau R. Cognitive science and survey methods. In: Jabine TB, Straf ML, Tanur JM and Tourangeau R (eds), Cognitive Aspects of Survey Methodology: Building a Bridge Between Disciplines. Washington, DC: National Academy Press, 1984;73—100.

UK National Case-control Study Group. Oral contraceptive use and breast cancer risk in young women. Lancet 1989;973—982.

Walker AM and Lanes SF. Misclassification of covariates. Stat Med 1991;10:1181—1196.

Walker AM and Blettner M. Comparing imperfect measures of exposure. Am J Epidemiol 1985;121:-783—790.

Walter SD and Irwig LM. Estimation of test error rates, disease prevalence and relative risk from misclassified data: a review. J Clin Epidemiol 1988;41:923—937.

Weinberg C. Towards a clearer definition of confounding. Amer J Epidemiol 1993;137:1—8.

Weinstock MA, Colditz GA, Willett WC, Stampfer MJ, Rosner B and Speizer FE. Recall (report) bias and reliability in the retrospective assessment of melanoma risk. Am J Epidemiol 1991;133:240—245.

Werler MM, Pober BR, Nelson K and Holmes LB. Reporting accuracy among mothers of malformed and nonmalformed infants. Am J Epidemiol 1989;129:415—421.

©1995 Elsevier Science B.V. All rights reserved.

Interpretation of epidemiologic studies with modestly elevated relative risks

Göran Pershagen

Institute of Environmental Medicine, Karolinska Institute, Stockholm, Sweden

Abstract. This article was presented at the Federal Focus Conference "The proper role of epidemiology in regulatory risk assessment" on October 13–14, 1994, at Lansdowne Conference Center, Virginia, USA.

Key words: bias, epidemiology, estimation, identification, methodology, risk.

Introduction

Epidemiologic evidence is increasingly used in risk assessment. When risks are substantial, such as lung cancer from tobacco smoking and some occupational exposures, there is generally little controversy in the interpretation of epidemiologic findings. However, when associations are weak, i.e., relative risks in the order of two or lower, the consequences of bias have to be assessed carefully. Most studies on risk factors in the general environment show only modestly elevated relative risks, but these effects may still be important from a public health point of view if large numbers of people are exposed.

The understanding of bias and its consequences is central in epidemiology. This is particularly important in the evaluation of epidemiologic evidence showing weak associations. The aim of this review is to discuss qualitative and quantitative implications of bias for the interpretation of epidemiologic studies with modestly elevated relative risks. Both risk identification and risk estimation will be addressed. Examples are primarily taken from studies on environmental causes of lung cancer, such as environmental tobacco smoke (ETS) and residential radon exposure. However, it is not the intention to comprehensively evaluate the scientific evidence on certain environmental exposures but to illustrate methodological problems in the interpretation of the data.

Role of bias

Several definitions of bias in epidemiologic studies have been proposed (Miettinen,

---

Address for correspondence: Göran Pershagen, Department of Epidemiology, Institute of Environmental Medicine, Karolinska Institute, Box 210, S–171, 77 Stockholm, Sweden. Tel.: +46-468-728-6400. Fax: +46-468-313-961.

1985; Rothman, 1986; Norell, 1992; Steineck and Ahlbom, 1992). The definition used here is based on the concept of the study base, i.e., the person-time experience in which an epidemiologic study is conducted (Miettinen, 1985). Consequently, bias is subdivided into selection, misclassification and confounding pertaining to the conditions in the study base (Norell, 1992). Since a longitudinal design generally provides the most conclusive epidemiologic evidence, the discussion is focused on cohort and case-control studies.

Selection

Bias may result from the selection of study subjects into an epidemiologic study. In most epidemiologic investigations all individuals cannot be followed up and classified in respect of disease. This can result in an over- or underestimation of the relative risk. For example, in a hospital-based case-control study on residential radon exposure and lung cancer it was indicated that only about half of the cases in the population were included (Svensson, 1988). Furthermore, the referral to the hospitals was in association with urbanization, which showed some relation to a residential radon level. A potential bias was avoided by the use of hospital controls experiencing a similar type of selection.

Particular problems arise in the selection of controls for case-control studies. Ideally controls should reflect the exposure situation in the study base (Miettinen, 1985). Controls may be sampled from the population or selected among hospital patients. It is generally easier to achieve representativeness for population controls, but the nonresponse is often higher than for hospital controls. Both hospitals and population controls are sometimes used in the same study (Pershagen et al., 1992), and findings are strengthened if results using either type of control group show consistency.

In retrospective studies of lung cancer, and other diseases with a high lethality, it is often impossible to obtain exposure information directly from the study subjects. To enhance comparability of the exposure information, deceased controls are sometimes used (Pershagen et al., 1987; Pershagen et al., 1994). If the exposures at interest affect mortality, a misrepresentation will result, leading to biased estimates of relative risks (McLoughlin et al., 1985). For example, smoking habits are overrepresented among dead controls, which gives rise to an underestimation of risks associated with smoking (Järup and Pershagen, 1991). If the only purpose is to control confounding from smoking, unbiased estimates of relative risks associated with other exposures may be achieved if these do not influence mortality (Howe, 1991). Overrepresentation of smoking among deceased controls is avid if those with smoking-related causes of death are excluded (Pershagen et al., 1994).

Misclassification

Most epidemiologic investigations suffer from misclassification of exposure and health effects. The measurements of exposure and health effects can be afflicted with random and systematic errors. Both types of error result in biased estimates of the relative risk. It is essential to assess how misclassification can affect the direction and magnitude of this bias.

Imprecise exposure data will generally lead to dilution effects, i.e., the association between exposure and disease is weakened (Armstrong, 1990). For example, in the studies on ETS and lung cancer the exposure data were obtained from interviews or questionnaires, and with few exceptions no validation of the information was attempted (EPA, 1992). The most common measure of exposure was spouses who smoked, which may be a more accurate predictor of ETS exposure for women than for men, where other sources predominate (Cummings et al., 1989; Sandler et al., 1989). It is clear, however, that there are many sources of ETS exposure which should be considered if the total exposure is to be assessed and that this depends also on cultural factors (Coughlin et al., 1989; Cummings et al., 1989; Riboli et al., 1990). On the other hand, the failure in some studies to obtain clearer associations between ETS exposure and lung cancer risk using more complex exposure models than smoking of spouses, may partly be explained by less reliable reporting of such exposures (Pron et al., 1988).

Attempts have been made to quantitatively assess the influence of nondifferential misclassification of exposure on the risk estimates for ETS and lung cancer (Wald et al., 1986). Using data on urinary cotinine excretion it is suggested that the relative risk comparing exposed with truly unexposed to ETS should be more in the order 1.5 if the observed relative risk comparing nonsmokers living with smokers and nonsmokers is 1.3. Only recent exposure was included in this calculation and the imprecision will be even greater if lifetime exposure is of importance.

Misclassification of exposure may also be differential between cases and controls. A difference in the quality of exposure data provided by cases and controls and is often referred to as recall bias. Some of the studies on ETS and lung cancer, which included deceased subjects, did not match on vital status in the selection of controls (EPA, 1992). As a rule, this led to a higher percentage of surrogate respondents for the cases because of the high lethality of lung cancer. Quality differences in the information on ETS exposure between index and surrogate respondents could result in biased estimates of the relative risks, however, one study suggests that this would be unimportant (Cummings et al., 1989).

Nondifferential misclassification of the health effects will also result in a dilution of the association. For example, secondary lung tumors and carcinomas with unknown primary site appeared in about one sixth of reported cases of lung cancer on death certificates in the USA (Garfinkel, 1981) and in central health registers in Sweden (Pershagen et al., 1987) among female nonsmokers. When rare diseases are studied the specificity of the measurement of disease is of greater importance for the attenuation effect than the sensitivity (Norell, 1992).

Confounding

Confounding is unlikely to explain relative risks in the order of two or higher (Axelson, 1978). However, an adequate control of confounding is crucial in epidemiologic studies with modestly elevated relative risks. In the studies on ETS and lung cancer probably the most important source of bias is confounding by unreported active smoking. There is a tendency for smokers to marry smokers, and in conjunction with some misclassification of smokers as nonsmokers this would tend to produce a spurious association between spouse smoking and lung cancer.

One crucial factor for estimation of the bias is the proportion of those classified as nonsmokers who actually have been smokers. Using biological markers of nicotine exposure it has been indicated that up to 3% of subjects classifying themselves as nonsmokers have levels consistent with regular smoking (Wald et al., 1986; Lee 1988; Riboli et al., 1990; Thompson et al., 1990). Studies involving multiple reports of smoking over several years as well as studies using surrogates suggest that in the order of about 5% of ever smokers may deny smoking (Lee, 1988). Several investigations indicate that surrogates can provide valid information to separate smokers from nonsmokers (Pershagen, 1984; McLoughlin et al., 1985; Metzner et al., 1989; U.S. Surgeon General, 1990; Nelson, et al., 1994), which makes this source of information useful for validation. Very limited and inconclusive data are available for smoking misclassification at interview with newly diagnosed lung cancer cases, which was the source of information in most epidemiological studies on ETS exposure and lung cancer.

A few attempts have been made to quantify the influence of confounding by smoking on the risk estimates for lung cancer in nonsmokers living with smokers. Using different assumption quite discrepant conclusions were reached. Wald et al. (1986) claimed that this source of bias would explain only about 15% of the observed risk, while Lee (1988) argued that most of the association was due to this factor. It is likely that the extent of smoking confounding bias differ between studies because of differences in smoking habits, risks associated with smoking and misclassification rates.

Negative confounding is probably as common as positive confounding, and also deserves attention in the interpretation of epidemiologic evidence. For example, negative confounding by smoking has been observed in studies on residential radon exposure and lung cancer (Létourneau, et al., 1994; Pershagen et al., 1994). This may lead to underestimation of the true effect or that no association is observed. Imprecision in the information on confounders, such as smoking habits, may give rise to residual confounding even if these factors are controlled in the analysis.

Risk identification

In general, it is not possible to draw conclusions on causality from a single epidemiologic study. This is particularly relevant if only weak associations were observed. Instead, the interpretation must rely on evidence from different sources, including animal experiments and other epidemiologic studies. The evaluation is facilitated if the findings are supported by knowledge regarding etiologic mechanisms. For example, the credibility of a causal relation between exposure to electromagnetic fields and cancer based on the epidemiologic observations, has been challenged in light of the lack of evidence on plausible mechanisms. On the other hand, cancer induction by low level exposure to tobacco smoke and radon progeny may be less unlikely.

In an effort to enhance statistical power, data from different epidemiologic studies are sometimes combined in meta- or pooled analyses. Meta-analyses use summary measures from different studies, such as point estimates of relative risk and variance, while individual data for each study subject are used in the pooled analysis (Friedenreich, 1993). Pooled analyses are generally more informative than meta-analyses, particularly in relation to the possibility for studies of subgroups.

It is questionable to what extent meta or pooled analyses of epidemiologic studies are useful for assessment of causality. For example, meta-analyses of the epidemiologic studies on ETS and lung cancer in nonsmokers clearly show that there is a statistically significant increase in the relative risk of about 20—30% (EPA, 1992; Lee, 1992). As indicated above, relative risks in this range may be explained by bias. An evaluation of qualitative and quantitative aspects of bias is thus central when causality is addressed in the interpretation. Unfortunately, important information on data quality and potential confounding factors is often lacking. Evidence of consistency between and within studies, such as exposure-response relationships facilitates the evaluation.

A meta-analysis may sometimes complicate the assessment of causality. It is difficult to adequately consider quality aspects of different studies in the combined analysis. Furthermore, there may be real differences in the exposure-response relation between studies because of interactions. For example, a recent pooled analysis of three studies on residential radon exposure and lung cancer showed no association (Lubin et al., 1994). However, two of the studies (from New Jersey and Stockholm) indicated a positive relation, but not the third study. This study was performed in Shenyang, China, where air pollution levels from both indoor and outdoor sources were extremely high, and this may have affected the radiation doses to the bronchial epithelium (James, 1988). There was no clear heterogeneity between the studies upon statistical testing, but these tests generally have a low power (Friedenrich, 1993).

In the interpretation of studies with modestly elevated relative risks it is essential to differentiate between inconclusive and negative evidence (Ahlbom et al., 1990). Several criteria have to be met if an investigation is to be interpreted as negative. The observed relative risk should lie close to unity, with a narrow confidence interval. This necessitates a large study base if exposure and/or disease occurrence is rare. Furthermore, the exposure information must have a high precision and negative confounding effects should be adequately controlled. It is difficult to fulfill these requirements at the same time, which means that conclusively negative epidemiologic studies are rare.

Using new developments in molecular biology it may be possible to enhance the

58

resolution power of epidemiologic studies. This can involve increased precision of the exposure information, enhanced specificity of outcome measures and identification of susceptible groups. For example, exposure to genotoxic agents can be monitored by measurements of DNA-adducts and mutations of marker genes, such as the hypoxantine—guanin—phosphoribosyltransfererase (hprt) gene (Hemminki et al., 1990, Tates et al., 1991). Furthermore, specific mutational patterns in genes involved in cancer induction, such as the p-53 tumor suppressor gene, may be more closely linked to certain exposures (Vähäkangas et al., 1992). Genetically determined variations in the ability to metabolize xenobiotics, could make it possible to focus on highly susceptible subgroups of the population in epidemiologic studies (Idle, 1991).

Risk estimation

When a causal association is considered credible, epidemiologic investigations are particularly useful for quantitative risk assessment. If studies are population-based the proportion of disease attributed to the exposure (etiologic fraction) may also be computed. This is essential for setting priorities in prevention, but should be used cautiously with due attention to the quality problems that affect epidemiologic evidence. However, the uncertainties are usually even greater when risk estimates are based on data in experimental animals.

In view of the difficulties in determining risks with high accuracy at low exposures in epidemiologic studies, risk estimation is sometimes based on extrapolation from high doses. For example, studies in miners have constituted the basis for quantitative risk assessment on residential radon exposure and lung cancer (NAS, 1988; ICRP, 1993). The linear relative risk model is used widely for risk estimation regarding carcinogens (EPA, 1983; WHO, 1987). It is supported to some extent by empirical data down to low doses for agents causing mutations (NAS, 1988). On the other hand, it may be more relevant to assume threshold effects for agents operating at other stages in the cancer induction process (Paustenbach, 1989). Risk estimation based on downward extrapolation is most uncertain at the lowest doses. The exposure to environmental agents is often skewed, such as for residential radon, which implies that the population attributable proportion is highly dependent on the estimates in the low exposure range.

Imprecision in the exposure estimation is likely to cause an attenuation of the exposure-response relation (Armstrong, 1990). If the precision of the method for exposure measurement is known it is possible to adjust the risk estimates for this bias. For example, there have been great efforts to assess the quality of different methods for dietary assessment in epidemiologic studies, and corrections have sometimes been performed of the risk estimates (Rosner et al., 1989). Unfortunately, the quality of most methods for exposure estimation is not known, which makes it difficult to adequately evaluate the degree of attenuation of the exposure-response relations.

A recent epidemiologic study from Sweden showed an increased lung cancer risk related to estimated time weighted residential radon exposure (Pershagen et al., 1994). The increase in risk per unit exposure appeared linear and multiplied the risk associated with smoking. Although great efforts were made to obtain detailed information on radon exposure, including measurements in close to 9,000 homes of the study subjects, it is clear that a substantial uncertainty remained in the exposure estimation. Several methods used to correct for imprecision in the exposure information indicated that the observed risks represented an underestimation of the true risk by a factor of about two. Obviously, this has profound effects on the risk assessment.

Conclusions

There is an inherent conflict between the demands from regulatory agencies as well as the general public for data enabling precise risk estimation and the information that science can deliver. Qualitative and quantitative risk assessment is often based on epidemiologic evidence showing modestly elevated relative risks, i.e., in the order of two or lower. Consequences of bias may be particularly deleterious for the interpretation of relative risks in this range. Important potential sources of bias include selection effects, misclassification and confounding.

Risk identification based on epidemiologic data with modestly elevated relative risks should focus more on quality aspects of the studies and less on statistical properties of the associations. Consequently, meta- or pooled analyses of different studies are of limited value in this respect. Evidence of internal consistency such as exposure-response relationships and coherence between studies is more important for the interpretation.

In evaluating epidemiologic investigations showing modestly elevated relative risks, it is essential to differentiate between inconclusive and negative studies, i.e., studies indicating no association between exposure and disease. Several criteria have to be met if a study is to be regarded as negative, including a large size and precise exposure data. Conclusively negative epidemiologic studies are rare.

When a causal association is considered credible, epidemiologic studies may be useful for quantitative risk assessment. Imprecision in the exposure estimation is likely to cause attenuation of the exposure-response relations, and may lead to substantial underestimation of attributable risks. Risk estimates can be adjusted for this bias if the precision of the exposure measures is known.

In view of the difficulties in determining risks with high accuracy at low exposures in epidemiologic studies, risk estimation is often based on extrapolation from high doses. Obviously, such risk estimates are most uncertain at the lowest doses. The uncertainty in the estimation of population attributable risks is aggravated because exposures to environmental agents are often skewed, with a large fraction of the population in the low dose range.

60

References

Ahlbom A, Axelson O, Stöttrup Hansen E, Hogstedt C, Jensen UJ and Olsen J. Interpretation of "negative" studies in occupational epidemiology. Scand J Work Environ Health 1990;16:153–157.

Armstrong B. The effects of measurement errors on relative risk regressions. Am J Epidemiol 1990; 132:1176–1184.

Axelson O. Aspects on confounding in occupational health epidemiology. Scand J Work Environ Health 1978;4:98–102.

Coughlin J, Hammond SK and Gann PH. Development of epidemiological tools for measuring environmental tobacco smoke exposure. Am J Epidemiol 1989;130:696–704.

Cummings KM, Markello SJ, Mahoney MC and Marshall JR. Measurement of lifetime exposure to passive smoke. Am J Epidemiol 1989;130:122–132.

EPA. Health assessment document for acrylonitrile. Washington DC: U.S. Environmental Protection Agency, DC, 1983.

EPA. Respiratory health effects of passive smoking: lung cancer and other disorders. Washington DC: U.S. Environmental Protection Agency, 1992.

Friedenreich CM. Methods for pooled analyses of epidemiologic studies. Epidemiology 1993;4:295–302.

Garfinkel L. Time trends in lung cancer mortality among nonsmokers and a note on passive smoking. J Natl Cancer Inst 1981;66:1061–1066.

Hemminki K, Grzybowska E, Chorazy M et al. DNA adducts in humans environmentally exposed to aromatic compounds in an industrial area of Poland. Carcinogenesis 1990;11:1229–1231.

Howe GR. Using dead controls to adjust for confounders in case-control studies. Am J Epidemiol 1991; 134:689–690.

Idle JR. Is environmental carcinogenesis modulated by host polymorphism? Mutation Res 1991;247:259.

International Commission on Radiological Protection. Protection against Radon–222 at home and at work. ICRP Publication 65. Ann ICRP 1993;23:1–45.

James AC. Radon and its decay products in indoor air. In: Nazaroff WW, Nero AV (eds) Lung Dosimetry. New York: John Wiley and Sons, 1988.

Järup L and Pershagen G. Arsenic exposure, smoking and lung cancer in smelter workers – a case-control study. Am J Epidemiol 1991;134:545–551.

Lee PN. Environmental Tobacco Smoke and Mortality. Basel: Karger, 1992.

Lee PN. Misclassification of Smoking Habits and Passive Smoking. Berlin: Springer, 1988.

Létourneau EG, Krewski D, Choi NW et al. A case-control study of residential radon and lung cancer in Winnipeg, Manitoba. Am J Epidemiol 1994;140:310–322.

Lubin JH, Liang Z, Hrubec Z et al. Radon exposure in residences and lung cancer among women: Combined analysis of three studies. Cancer Causes Control 1994;5:114–128.

McLoughlin JK, Dietz MS, Mehl ES and Blot WJ. Reliability of surrogate information on cigarette smoking by type of informant. Am J Epidemiol 1985;126:144–146.

Metzner HL, Lamphiear DE, Thompson FE, Oh MS and Hawthorne VM. Comparison of surrogate and subject reports of dietary practices, smoking habits and weight among married couples in the Tecumseh diet methodology study. J Clin Epidemiol 1989;42:367–375.

Miettinen OS. Principles of Occurrence Research in Medicine. New York: John Wiley and Sons, 1985.

National Academy of Sciences. Radon and other internally deposited alpha-emitters. BEIR IV. Washington DC: National Academy Press, 1988.

Nelson LM, Longstreth WT, Koepsell TD, Checkoway H and van Belle G. Completeness and accuracy of interview data from proxy respondents: demographic, medical and lifestyle factors. Epidemiology 199;45:204–217.

Norell S. A Short Course in Epidemiology. New York: Raven Press, 1992.

Paustenbach DJ. Important recent advances in the practice of health risk assessment: implications for the 1990s. Regul Toxicol Pharmacol 1989;10:204–243.

Pershagen G. Validity of questionnaire data on smoking and other exposures, with special reference to environmental tobacco smoke. Eur J Resp Dis 1984;65:76–80.

Pershagen G, Hrubec Z and Svensson C. Passive smoking and lung cancer in Swedish women. Am J Epidemiol 1987;125:17–24.

Pershagen G, Liang ZH, Hrubec Z, Svensson C and Boice JD Jr. Residential radon exposure and lung cancer in women. Health Phys 1992;63:179–186.

Pershagen G, Åkerblom G, Axelson O et al. Residental radon exposure and lung cancer in Sweden. N Engl J Med 1994;330:159–164.

Pron GE, Burch DJ, Howe GR and Miller AB. The reliability of passive smoking histories reported in a case-control study of lung cancer. Am J Epidemiol 1988;127:267–284.

Riboli E, Preston-Martin S, Saracci R et al. Exposure of nonsmoking women to environmental tobacco smoke: a ten-country collaborative study. Cancer Causes Control 1990;1:243–252.

Rosner B, Willett WC and Spiegelman D. Correction of logistic regression relative risk estimates and confidence intervals for systematic within-person measurement error. Stat Med 1989;8:1051–1069.

Rothman KJ. Modern epidemiology. Boston: Little, Brown and Company, 1986.

Sandler DP, Helsing KJ, Comstock GW and Shore DL. Factors associated with past household exposure to tobacco smoke. Am J Epidemiol 1989;129:380–387.

Steineck G and Ahlbom A. A definition of bias founded on the concept of the study base. Epidemiology 1992;3:477–482.

Svensson C. Lung cancer etiology in women. Stockholm: Karolinska Institutet Ph.D. thesis, 1988.

Tates AD, Grummt T, Törnqvist M et al. Biological and chemical monitoring of occupational exposure to ethylene oxide. Mutation Res 1991;250:483–497.

Thompson SG, Stone R, Nanchahal K and Wald NJ. Relation of urinary cotinine concentrations to cigarette smoking and to exposure to other people's smoke. Thorax 1990;45:356–361.

U.S. Surgeon General. The health benefits of smoking cessation. Washington DC: United States Department of Health and Human Services, 1990.

Wald NJ, Nanchahal K, Thompson SG and Cuckle HS. Does breathing other people's tobacco smoke cause lung cancer? Br Med J 1986;293:1217–1222.

World Health Organization. Air quality guidelines for Europe. European series No 23. Copenhagen: WHO Regional Office for Europe, 1987.

Vähäkangas KH, Samet JM, Metcalf RA et al. Mutations of p53 and ras genes in radon-associated lung cancer from uranium miners. Lancet 1992;339:576-579.

©1995 Elsevier Science B.V. All rights reserved.
The Role of Epidemiology in Regulatory Risk Assessment
J.D. Graham, editor.

Behavioral factors affecting the interpretation of weak associations in epidemiology

Linda C. Koo

Cancer Research Laboratory, Nam Long Hospital, Hong Kong

Key words: assessment, association, behaviour, design, epidemiology, risk.

Introduction

Although epidemiological data on humans are important in supplementing results from animal studies for risk assessment, the interpretation of epidemiological studies and their applicability for establishing statutory regulations on human exposures must be done with awareness of some of the underlying influential factors that may affect research results. These factors may be especially pertinent where the estimated relative risks are low but public concern about these exposures are high. This may result in data which are more open to selection and interpretation by the researcher, design biases and weaknesses, behavioral correlates of the risk factor, and confounders which may not be controllable by statistical adjustment. I shall be commenting on these underlying behavioral issues from the perspective of an epidemiologist with anthropological training who has been conducting research on lung cancer, air pollution, diet, and respiratory diseases.

Unlike some of the classical studies on such powerful agents like active smoking and lung cancer (e.g., Wynder and Graham, 1950) where dose-response effects would result however one measured exposure (number of cig/day, number years smoked, age started, etc.), wherever it was done, and regardless of small imperfections in design and conduct, epidemiological studies on low risk agents are more vulnerable to weaknesses in research design and human behavioral responses. These problems are magnified when studying the epidemiology of chronic diseases like cardiovascular disease or cancers of solid organs because of their long latency periods. For retrospective studies, questionnaire design is important to help subjects recall past exposures and how they have changed over their lifetime. However, there must be some understanding of how these results may be influenced by current attitudes and motives of both the researchers and the researched.

In discussing the behavioral issues that might affect the interpretation of low risk agents identified in epidemiological research, my comments shall be directed at: 1)

Address for correspondence: Linda Koo, Cancer Research Laboratory, 7th Floor, Nam Long Hospital, 30 Nam Long Shan Road, Wong Chuk Hang, Hong Kong. Tel.: +852–552–7923. Fax: +852–817–6528.

the political climate and public attitudes; 2) characteristics of the researcher; 3) research design; 4) subjects studied; 5) analyses that are done; and 6) results that are published.

Political climate and public attitudes

"No man is an island" is an axiom that has subtle influences in all phases of epidemiologic research. Unlike laboratory animals, human beings — be they epidemiologists, patient-cases, neighborhood controls, reviewers, publishers, fundors, or regulators — are influenced by prevailing attitudes and beliefs. With an active media publicizing news on the latest health hazard, everyone is "contaminated" to some extent. Thus the usual assumption that epidemiologic research is conducted in a value free "objective" environment is rarely achieved. Its resulting influence on epidemiological results shall be discussed below.

Characteristics of the researcher

The underlying beliefs and attitudes of a researcher may influence the kinds of questions that are asked (and not asked) in a research project, how the questions are asked (especially if they will be conducting the interviews), whether unexpected results will be pursued, and the selection of data for publication.

In the current controversies surrounding the health effects of environmental tobacco smoke (ETS) many examples can be found. Slattery et al. (1989) found that ETS is a risk factor for cervical cancer. Yet, as commented by Zang et al. (1989), the authors failed to gather data about the number of sexual partners their mates had, whether they visited bars and discos (where there is much ETS and promiscuity), the age when sexual behavior began, their previous history of sexually transmitted diseases, etc. Instead of asking about some of known risk factors for cervical cancer, as there is evidence that it is a sexually transmitted disease associated with certain variants of the human papillomaviruses or herpes simplex 2 viruses, their data gathering ignored such risk factors and focused on active and passive smoking, where there is little evidence of biological plausibility.

Similarly, in another study associating the mother's exposure to ETS during pregnancy and resulting low birth weights in infants (Martin and Bracken, 1986), no data were gathered on maternal nutrition except alcohol, although maternal malnutrition is a well known risk factor for underweight full-term newborns (Williams and Jelliffe, 1972). Especially as the authors noted that the ETS exposed mothers were more likely to be young, single, nonwhite, and poorly educated, the association of these attributes with poor nutrition is highly likely.

Perhaps one of the more recognized influences on the researcher is the source of funding. Many publishers now require that research funding and other financial interests in the outcome of a study be declared. This is open recognition that a researcher's motives and attitudes may influence a study's results.

Many epidemiologists also have personal and political goals to fight against smoking, drinking, guns, occupational hazards, nuclear radiation, pesticides, etc. which may affect the kinds of research they do and how they present it. This is particularly true among health researchers because there is self-selection in choice of occupations. With these emotional investments, many find it difficult to accept that low doses of some risk factors may have negligible or even beneficial outcomes (e.g., drinking and heart disease). Or, that some agents may be associated with decreased risk, e.g., cancer of the endometrium and Parkinsonism is described in the IARC report on Tobacco Smoking as "disease for which excess mortality in nonsmokers may be preventable by smoking" (IARC 1985:40).

Consequently, the influence of a researcher's attitudes and beliefs, although nebulous to specify, may play a larger role in interpretations of weak associations in epidemiology than in situations where there is a stronger cause-effect relationship. As stated by Florey (1988), some of the interpretations "may reflect more the authors' points of view or degree of scientific caution" than scientific plausibility.

Research design

When an environmental risk factor commands much public interest, e.g., radiation from nuclear power plants, pesticides in food, radon in homes, etc. there is a bandwagon effect stimulating others to conduct research and obtain results as fast as possible. With this rush, especially for weak risk agents, the underlying strategy is frequently the more, the faster, the better. If more subjects are studied, statistical power is improved so the results will be more "significant". Consequently data from surrogates will be used as substitutes for true subjects, mailed questionnaires or telephone interviews will replace face-to-face interviews, or information on lifestyles or exposures will be gathered from patient files. The poorer data gathering methods are cheaper and less labor intensive to do. However, as an example, from our worldwide survey on published studies of smoking histories among lung cancer patients, the use of surrogates, patient records, or mailed questionnaires always produced lower reported percentages of smokers than personal interview studies (Koo and Ho, 1990).

It is difficult to put a quantitative weight onto qualitative differences between studies, especially as studies with larger numbers seem more impressive. One must realize, however, that given the limited energy of researchers and interobserver variation, it is highly likely that the larger the numbers studied, the poorer the quality control.

For the researcher, there are also few noticeable benefits for the much larger expenditure of time and energy necessary for top quality data. After all, reputations are based on publications, and larger numbers of studied subjects carry more weight in meta-analysis. Although it may be argued that poorer data gathering methods will also generate more noise which will cancel out any observed effects, they may also exaggerate biases and give statistical significance to results which are due to poor research design.

For epidemiological research in non-Western countries, there is often over or under emphasis on local customs and behaviors. For non-Western researchers who have been trained in Western scientific methods, there is a tendency to do "copycat" research to see if the same risk factor exerts similar effects in their society. Many do not take sufficient account of the local adjustments in research design necessary to assess how different behavioral factors or other exposures peculiar to their local community may be associated with the exposure that is studied. For example, from our Hong Kong studies, we have identified through personal monitoring and home monitoring studies that the major source of indoor air pollution in homes is incense, and not ETS (Koo et al., 1990, Koo et al., 1994), although ETS is the "most ubiquitous indoor air pollutant" in the USA (EPA 1992). For non-Western countries, these design inadequacies are sometimes not helped by research funding from Western countries. The Western fundors usually have little knowledge of local conditions, and the outside funds may exert subtle pressures on local researchers to find similar or positive results. Alternatively, at the other extreme, there are epidemiological studies in non-Western countries which have tried to explain certain common diseases as being primarily due to some unique exposure specific to that culture (e.g kerosene stove fumes and lung cancer by Leung, 1977). Usually, this is only plausible if the disease exhibits unusual patterns (e.g., age-specific incidence, histological type, clinical progression of the disease, etc.) in that culture.

Subjects studied

Some of the weaknesses in epidemiological studies come from biases due to a lack of understanding of the behaviors and attitudes of the study subjects. We can classify such factors as internal beliefs and behaviors, behavioral traits among cases, such factors among controls, and the effect of the observer on the observed.

Most of the activities that humans do have underlying reasons, and when certain traits are shared, some predictable behaviors will result. This is why if one knows the basic demographic profile of a person e.g., his age, gender, race, education, residence, and occupation, we can generally predict the likelihood of other behaviors, like tendency to smoke, drink, be obese, take drugs, etc. However, in epidemiological studies, we treat these variables as "independent" and somehow assume that we can "control" these variables statistically.

Additionally, the interrelationships of different behavioral traits may not be obvious. For example, in our previous study of diet and lung cancer risk among nonsmoking Hong Kong Chinese women, smaller household sizes were significantly associated with higher risk (Koo, 1988). From another angle, increasing parity among the women also significantly reduced their risk for lung cancer. These data seemed to point to the possibility that the physiological changes associated with pregnancy somehow increased bodily protective factors or the immune system. However, further analyses of the data indicated that smaller households significantly consumed fresh vegetables and fish less often than larger ones, and these dietary patterns were associated with increased risk for lung cancer in this population. One therefore wonders whether other research findings whereby female fecundity has been identified as a risk factor (e.g., breast or colon cancer) is also reflecting the dietary consequences of larger family sizes rather than the physiological changes associated with childbirth.

As commented by Samet (1991:349) epidemiological studies can illustrate "the difficulty of fully disentangling the correlated dimensions of human behavior that determine disease risk" and for example, "It is unlikely that confounding by lifestyle correlates of smoking can be fully controlled by simply including indicator variables in multivariate models." Yet, most of the time, that is how data on subject's attributes are treated in epidemiological studies.

The attitudes of a sick person will also be different from one who is well, especially if the sick person has a life-threatening disease. In case-control studies where characteristics of the two groups are compared, the recall of a patient about their past exposures will tend to be thought through in more detail than that of a healthy population control. In Fontham et al.'s study (1991) on ETS and lung cancer where they used both colon cancer patients and healthy people as controls, the odds ratios from ETS exposure when patient controls were used was always lower than when population controls were used.

It is also inevitable that sick people will think about their disease, and have a lay explanation for the causative factors for their sickness. From lay conceptions, patients with respiratory disease will try to attribute it to inhaled factors, and those with stomach or intestinal problems with ingestants. This is encouraged by the fact that in the prodromal stages of their disease, they may be more sensitive to inhaled or ingested agents respectively. Thus epidemiological studies looking at weak exposures may be actually reflecting these lay conceptions and sensitivities.

When surrogates are used for data collection, an even more complex mixture of lay beliefs and familial relationships and motives may be reflected in the data collected. In Garfinkel et al.'s (1985) study of ETS and lung cancer risk by identity of the case-respondent, relative risks were lower when the surrogate respondent was the husband of the patient and higher when they were the child of the patient.

Additionally, when healthy controls are interviewed, they have less motivation to expend the mental energy needed to recall about exposure than cases. This is especially true when collecting data about the distant past. These problems of recall bias are further exaggerated when impersonal methods like telephone interviews or mailed questionnaires are conducted on the controls, and face-to-face personal interviews are conducted on the patient cases. The latter are frequently lying in hospital with much time on their hands and it is well known that response and compliance rates are higher for patients than normal people. It is therefore to be expected that patient cases will tend to recall more exposures, especially those which they believe are related to their illness.

The effects of the observer on the observed may also influence research results.

This is particularly true for the "compliant" patient cases. Also, if an interviewer knows the hypothesis being tested, borderline situations may be given a higher or lower grading, questions may be asked in a particular way, nonverbal communication may be different, and the degree of probing may differ between patients and controls. This problem of interviewer bias may be somewhat minimized by comparing patient cases with patient controls, and a large number of possible hypothesis are tested in the original design of the study, but it is almost impossible to blind interviewers about the status of a patient vs. a healthy population control. Of course, using patient controls introduces other problems of confounding and bias because their underlying environmental, behavioral, physiological, or psychological traits may be similar or antagonistic to the situation among the cases.

Analyses of data

In studying weak associations in epidemiology, it is even more important that the results of multiple methods of assessing an exposure are consistent in showing increased risk to reduce the effects of biases and confounders. As an example, we attempted to do this in a retrospective case-control study evaluating past ETS exposures in Hong Kong (Koo et al., 1984; Koo et al., 1987). Utilizing the person-place-time model in epidemiology, we assessed exposure by who smokes (relationship to subject), how many people smoked, what they smoked, how much they smoked, and the duration of each exposure from each smoker; where ETS exposure occurred (home, work, elsewhere); and what period in life ETS exposure occurred (childhood, adulthood, current). We then summarized the exposures from multiple smokers, places, and times in terms of hours, years, and total numbers of cigarettes of exposure to estimate lifetime doses. From these multiple angles of looking at ETS exposure, we did not find dose-response effects.

The possibility of confounders affecting weak associations in epidemiology is the subject of much debate. There are at least two issues involved: identifying the confounders (which entails an understanding of the behavioral dynamics linking the associations), and taking account of the confounders in data analysis. Neither is easy to do. Although epidemiologists utilize logistic regression models to "control" the effects of variables which they believe are possible confounders, the results are still imperfect and much data can be lost.

An example is shown in Table 1 where lung cancer relative risks (RR) from incense exposure are shown. We have compared RR estimations by looking at all subjects and controlling the influence of smoking by lifetime tobacco amount or whether they ever-smoked (+/–), and also by separate analyses of nonsmokers and smokers. The comparison shows that in a mixed population of smokers and nonsmokers, the lower risk associated with incense exposure among the smokers is not apparent, even when there is statistical adjustment for smoking. Therefore relationships which just affect one subgroup in an analysis may be obscured when analyzing a mixed population.

Table 1. Incense exposure and lung cancer relative risk (RR) among ever-married Hong Kong Chinese females.

	Years exposed to incense			
	0	1–39 (95% CI)	40–70 (95% CI)	Trend p value
Never smoked				
No. of cases/no. of controls	21/31	35/52	30/35	
Unadjusted RR[a]	1.00	1.07 (0.50–2.30)	0.98 (0.45–2.11)	0.99
Adjusted RR[b]	1.00	1.01 (0.45–2.26)	0.96 (0.41–2.27)	0.68
Ever smoked				
No. of cases/no. of controls	24/12	27/16	52/33	
Unadjusted RR[a]	1.00	0.47 (0.14–1.56)	0.27 (0.09–0.82)	0.01
Adjusted RR[c]	1.00	0.55 (0.11–2.82)	0.17 (0.03–0.81)	0.01
All				
No. of cases/no. of controls	45/43	62/68	82/86	
Unadjusted RR[a]	1.00	0.80 (0.46–1.41)	0.80 (0.46–1.39)	0.51
Adjusted RR[d]	1.00	0.93 (0.48–1.81)	0.67 (0.35–1.31)	0.35
Adjusted RR[e]	1.00	0.79 (0.41–1.51)	0.58 (0.31–1.12)	0.19

Source: 1981–1983 case control study as in Koo et al. (1987). [a]N:M matched analysis using PECAN, a conditional regression software package. [b]Adjusting for age ($\leq$60, 61–65, 66+), no. live births ($\leq$2, 3–5, 6+), birth place (HK or Macau +/–) and schooling (+/–). [c]Adjusted same as for [b] plus lifetime tabacco ($\leq$54.7, 54.71–100, 100.01–200, > 200 kg). [d]Adjusted same as for [b] plus lifetime tabacco amount (0, $\leq$54.7, 54.71–100, 100.01–200, > 200 kg). [e]Adjusted as for [b] plus ever smoked.

This example is also interesting because it shows that increasing doses of an air pollutant resulted in significantly reduced risk for lung cancer in smokers. In further analyses, we found that since incense burning is done for ancestor worship and this would be a behavior indicative of traditional lifestyles, incense burning was correlated with a traditional diet (e.g., more fresh fish and less alcohol) which was previously associated with reduced lung cancer risk in this population (Koo, 1988).

This example also shows the limitations of statistical adjustment, the difficulties in identifying confounders, and the problems with correlated behaviors which may not be disentangled by statistics. It is therefore probably advisable that when studying behaviors that are correlated, e.g., smokers tend to drink, an ethnic group tends to eat certain foods, or the whole range of behaviors and exposures correlated with gender and socio-economic status, that statistical analysis be done separately for the different groups to better understand the interweaving dynamics of behavior and exposure.

The preconceived beliefs and attitudes of a researcher are also important in data analysis. When results come as expected, it is generally human nature not to double check or do further analysis. Hence, the irony about reliability of data is that usually only unexpected results will have been double checked so that unexpected results are probably more reliable than expected ones. The possible biases introduced by a data analyzer is probably better recognized in the methodology of clinical trials, where the gold standard is a triple-blinded study, i.e., the data analyzer does not know who was or was not exposed.

Published results

Although it is well-known among all researchers who have tried to submit papers for publication (and for reviewers) that the possibility of negative data being accepted for publication is less than that for positive data, there are also other forces at work which influence what is in the published domain.

Due to constraints of space and also the desire of researchers to show positive results, sometimes published results only show those measurements where there were increased relative risks, and not those where no increases were found. There may not even be mention in the text that no results were found for some measurements of the exposure. This would result in the risk factor looking more strongly positive than it really is.

We know that this is a factor in some of the ETS studies. Perhaps when regulators want to assess research results on weak associations in epidemiology, they should go beyond what is published and inquire into all the data that were collected on the risk factor in a particular study to understand where there were insignificant results between exposure and risk.

Researchers may also not describe in a publication where they had contradictory or inconsistent results — the easier thing is to forget about those difficulties, especially with the pressure to get manuscripts published. Who would know? Why create criticisms from the reviewers? So contrary data and explanations are less likely to be found in a manuscript because authors generally want their research results to look more consistent.

Conclusion

Unlike interpretations of data from animal studies where possible confounders can be controlled by experimental design, and the experiment can be replicated by other researchers, in epidemiology we usually do not have the luxury of being able to control our human subjects. Our experimental laboratory is the world where different beliefs, practices, and environments provide variations in behaviors and exposures. For weak associations in epidemiology, it is important that similar risk estimates are obtained from similar exposures in a variety of cultures at different stages of economic development. This could help ensure that behavioral correlates and other confounders that may be operating in one culture or associated with a particular socio-economic class does not independently explain the health effects of the exposure under study.

Results from weak associations in epidemiology are also more vulnerable to a large number of personal factors among the researchers and the researched. Although not necessarily deliberate, the aims and motivations of researchers and subjects may introduce biases which may distort the putative association between exposure and risk. These problems are not necessarily neutralized by utilizing sophisticated statistical methods to control for possible confounders because this implies an understanding of what those confounders are and how they are related to the exposure under study. This may not be obvious. Furthermore, the use of meta-analysis to combine weak results from several studies may only serve to make statistically significant some of the research weaknesses that we have identified.

It is also important that reviewers of epidemiologic studies realize that there are many imperfections in any study in all its phases. An understanding of such weaknesses would be better understood if some of the reviewers have had actual experience in doing that type of research, including methodological design, logistics, questionnaire design, attempting to get funding, interviewing patients and controls, doing data analysis, writing the reports, and trying to get the manuscript published.

To maintain our professional credibility, and being wary of scientific fads, media publicity, and the pressures of lobbyists, epidemiologists and reviewers should be more cautious with risk factors where there are weak relative risks. After all, we shall be judged by time.

References

Environmental Protection Agency. Respiratory health effects of passive smoking: lung cancer and other disorders. Washington DC: EPA. 1992.

Florey CDV. Weak associations in epidemiological research: some examples and their interpretation. Int J Epidemiol 1988;17:950–954.

Fontham ETH, Correa P, Wu-Williams A, Reynolds P, Greenberg RS, Buffler PA, Chen VW, Boyd P, Alterman T, Austin DF, Liff J and Greenberg SD. Lung cancer in nonsmoking women: A multicenter case-control study. Cancer Epidemiol. Biomarkers Prev 1991;1:35–43.

Garfinkel L, Auerbach O and Joubert L. Involunatry smoking and lung cancer: a case-control study. J Natl Cancer Inst 1985;75:463–469.

International Agency for Research on Cancer. IARC Monographs on the evaluation of the carcinogenic risk of chemicals to humans, tobacco smoking. Vol 38. Lyon: IARC 1985.

Koo LC, Ho JH-C and Saw D. Is passive smoking an added risk factor for lung cancer in Chinese women? J Exp Clin Cancer Res 1984;3:277–283.

Koo LC, Ho JH-C, Saw D and Ho C-Y. Measurements of passive smoking and estimates of lung cancer risk among nonsmoking Chinese females. Int J Cancer 1987;39:162–169.

Koo LC. Dietary habits and lung cancer risk among Chinese females in Hong Kong who never smoked. Nutr Cancer 1988;11:155–172.

Koo LC, Ho JH-C, Ho C-Y, Matsuki H, Shimizu H, Mori T and Tominaga S. Personal exposure to nitrogen dioxide and its association with respiratory illness in Hong Kong. Am Rev Resp Dis 1990;141:1119–1126.

Koo LC and Ho JH-C. Worldwide epidemiological patterns of lung cancer in nonsmokers. Int J Epidemiol 1990;19:S14–S23.

Koo LC, Matsushita H, Ho JH-C, Wong MC, Shimizu H, Mori T, Matsuki and Tominaga S. Carcinogens in the indoor air of Hong Kong homes: levels, sources, and ventilation effects on seven polynuclear aromatic hyudrocarbons. Environ Technol 1994; 15:401–418.

Leung JSM. Cigarette smoking, the kerosene stove and lung cancer in Hong Kong. Br J Dis Chest 1977;

71:273–276.

Martin TR and Bracken MB. Association of low birth weight with passive smoke exposure in pregnancy. Am J Epidemiol 1986;124:633–642.

Samet JM. Editorial commentary: New effects of active and passive smoking on reproduction? Am J Epidemiol 1991;33:348–350.

Slattery ML, Robison LM, Schuman KL, Freench TK, Abbott TM, Overall JC and Gardner JW. Cigarettes smoking and exposure to passive smoke are risk factor for cervical cancer. J Am Med Assoc 1989;261:1593–1598.

Williams CD and Jelliffe DB. Mother and Child Health. London: Oxford University Press, 1972.

Wynder EL and Graham EA. Tobacco smoking as a possible etiological factor in bronchiogenic carcinoma. J Am Med Assoc 1950;143;329–336.

Zang EA, Wynder EL and Harris RE. Exposure to cigarette smoke and cervical cancer. Letter to the editor. J Am Med Assoc 1989;262:499.

©1995 Elsevier Science B.V. All rights reserved.
The Role of Epidemiology in Regulatory Risk Assessment
J.D. Graham, editor.

Epidemiology of weak associations

Ernst L. Wynder
American Health Foundation, New York, New York, USA

Key words: associations, confounders, education, epidemiology, smoking.

When determining causation in epidemiology, an odds ratio of 1.2 may have public health significance, particularly when involving a sizable proportion of the population. However, the issue is, that epidemiological biases need to be considered of whether in fact this odds ratio is artefactual.

The issue is that there are at least five different factors, including a selection of cases and controls and the consideration of biases, confounders, subgroup analysis, and the meaningfulness of logistic regression analysis, that can adversely affect, either positively or negatively, causative influences. While any of these factors alone may not account for an established weak association to be real, it is often the case that all of these factors can have some impact. For instance, we often see that the cases are interviewed directly, whereas the controls are interviewed by telephone. Whereas all the controls being alive speak for themselves, among cases, some of them have deceased, and hence it is surrogates who are interviewed. It is not always considered to what extent these different approaches towards cases and controls can influence a relative risk. In general, no-one would like to think that a case with a given disease looks at a question pertaining to that disease from a different vantage point than the control who has no relationship to this factor, particularly when asked about it on the telephone.

Confounders represent a particular problem since two major confounders, cigarette smoking and education, affect so many studies. Often we see that the cases are less educated than the controls, and although it is usually clear that an adjustment has to be made, one wonders how carefully this has to be done, particularly when many other variables are being adjusted simultaneously. Active smoking is, of course, a major confounder as shown in Fig. 1 (Berger and Wynder, 1994). In our studies we have shown that the total tobacco exposure in an individual's lifetime involving duration, number of cigarettes, brand of cigarettes has a broad impact on such wide ranging issues as diet and education. Most studies do not have such detailed data, on active tobacco smoking, available. If there is a smoker in a given household (Berger and Wynder, 1994), it is likely that the intake of dietary fat is positively affected, and

---

Address for correspondence: Ernst L. Wynder, American Health Foundation, 320 East 43rd Street, New York, NY 10017, USA. Tel.: +1-212-953-1900. Fax: +1-914-592-6317.

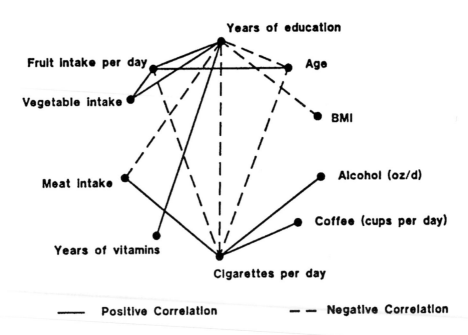

Fig. 1. Partial correlation structure of 10 variables for 3,810 men, from data collected by trained interviewers with a standardized questionnaire in eight hospitals in four cities (Chicago, Detroit, New York and Philadelphia) from 1985–1990 (U.S. Health Dept. of Health, Education and Welfare, Public Health Service, 1964). Source: AHF, 1991.

so one needs to consider this dietary factor as one contemplates causation. In a study on long-distance truck drivers, for instance, we have shown that this group smokes more, and eats more fatty foods because these individuals eat at truck stops, most of the time, and they serve these types of fatty foods more than the general population (Wynder and Miller, 1988). The combined effect of heavy smoking and high dietary fat intake can, therefore, account for the reported higher risk for cancer of the lung and bladder among long-distance truck drivers. In fact, our data has shown that proper adjustment for tobacco alone can eliminate the risk for long-distance truckers (Boffetta et al., 1989).

Tobacco as a confounder has not always generally been given the proper study in lung cancer among railway workers. Here in a recent review, we have shown that virtually none of the retrospective studies, except those conducted by our group, have had sufficient data on lifelong tobacco exposure to undertake the proper adjustment (Wynder and Higgins, 1986). Confounding, therefore, needs to be critically assessed as we contemplate causation, particularly in studies involving weak associations.

Bias is of particular concern because it is almost impossible to measure accurately. In our recent studies on dietary fat intake and breast cancer, we have observed that over the years, women with breast cancer report a lower and lower intake of dietary fat (Chlebowski et al., 1993). This situation is probably equivalent to that of the truck drivers, who have reported excessive diesel exhaust exposure and lung cancer patients reporting excessive exposure to the smoke of others, as being a part of human nature to blame someone or something else rather than ourselves. In respect to exposure to environmental tobacco smoke (ETS), particularly in recent years, with smoking so generally regarded as detrimental to our health, it has been shown that even current smoking, which could be verified by cotinine measurements, is misclassified by 1% to 3% of the population. It could, therefore, be assumed that long-term ex-smoking has an important higher rate of misclassification. In fact, a study by Heller, of individuals participating in the MONICA project showed a long-term misclassification rate as high as 15% (Heller et al.). Here, we need to note that the risk of lung cancer among long-term quitters never reaches the low level of those who have never smoked.

A good example of bias is the estimation of height and weight among individuals. Others and ourselves have shown that men tend to overestimate their height and women to underestimate their weight (Stewart et al., 1987). We suppose such biases to be a part of human nature and, in fact, are of a systematic nature, so that meta-analysis would not be helpful.

Subgroup analysis: All of us, as we undertake a study would do a variety of subgroup analyses that are increasingly made possible by the advance of computerization. Who is to know how many analyses we have done, and is it not likely, since we as investigators are also human, that we prefer to report those analyses that are positive and are less likely to report negative analyses? This investigator bias translates itself also into a publication bias in that journals and reviewers prefer to see positive studies published and that in fact many investigators with negative findings do not see the need to submit them for publication in the first place.

We need to consider logistic regression analysis. With the advent of software packages, we see all types of analyses being performed, such as, let us say, 60 cases and controls, which the investigators report they have simultaneously adjusted for analysis. In such analysis, one wonders how many cells were indeed blank. Here we are testing the technique of logistic regression analysis to its very limits.

In summary, all of these variables need to be considered as we contemplate causation. As we examine this issue, we need to recognize that while the industry-connected individual has a bias that the product of the company is not harmful the academic investigator has a bias towards positive findings. What we should do here is reflect on the Bradford Hill principles of causation, which we are listing again in Table 1, that were used as criteria of judgement in the first Surgeon General report on Smoking and Health in 1964 (U.S. Dept. of Health, Education and Welfare, Public Health Service, 1964), and in fact, were used by us in a 1954 paper on tobacco smoking as the cause and effect of lung cancer (Wynder, 1954), but are rarely used by investigators reporting on weak associations, which they deem to be causative. I would conclude that, as we contemplate causation in respect to weak associations in epidemiology, we carefully examine all the issues we have raised here, and then we determine the extent to which they fit with the criteria of judgement before we issue our own judgement as to whether a causative relationship indeed exists.

76

Table 1. Criteria for judgement of the casual significance of an association.

a. The consistency of the association
b. The strength of the association
c. The specificity of the association
d. The temporal relationship of the association
e. The coherence of the association

From the U.S. Dept. of Health, Education and Welfare, Public Health Service, 1964.

References

Berger J and Wynder EL. The correlation of epidemiological variables. J Clin Epidemiol 1994;47:941–952.

Boffetta F, Harris RE and Wynder EL. Diesel exhaust exposure and lung cancer risk. Exp Pathol 1989; 37:32–38.

Chlebowski RT, Blackburn GL, Buzzard IM et al. Adherence to a dietary fat intake reduction program in postmenopausal women receiving therapy for early breast cancer. J Clin Oncol 1993;11:2072–2080.

Heller WD, Sennewald E, Gostomzyk JG et al. Validation of ETS-exposure in a representative population in southern Germany, vol. 3, pp. 361–365, Helsinki, Finland.

Stewart AW, Jackson RT, Ford MA et al. Underestimation of relative weight by use of self-reported height and weight. Am J Epidemiol 1987;125;122–126.

U.S. Dept. of Health, Education and Welfare, Public Health Service. Smoking and Health. Report of the Advisory Committee To the Surgeon General of the Public Health Service. Washington DC: U.S. Govt. Printing Office (PHS Publ No. 1103), 1964.

Wynder EL. Tobacco as a cause of lung cancer: with special reference to the infrequency of lung cancer among nonsmokers. Penn Med J 1954;57:1073–1083.

Wynder EL and Higgins ITT. Exposure to diesel exhaust emissions and the risk of lung and bladder cancer. In: Ishiniski N, Koizuma A, Mclellan RD, Stober W (eds) Carcinogenic and Mutagenic Effects of Diesel Engine Exhaust, 1986.

Wynder EL and Miller S. Correspondence re Silverman DT et al. Motor exhaust-related occupation and bladder cancer. Cancer Res 1988;48:1989–1990.

©1995 Elsevier Science B.V. All rights reserved.
The Role of Epidemiology in Regulatory Risk Assessment
J.D. Graham, editor.

When and how to combine results from multiple epidemiological studies in risk assessment

Suresh H. Moolgavkar

Fred Hutchinson Cancer Research Center, Division of Public Health Sciences, Seattle, Washington, USA

Key words: carcinogen, epidemiology, heterogeneity, meta-analysis, potency, risk assessment.

Let me begin with a disclaimer. The title of this paper gives the impression that I will provide a recipe for determining when epidemiologic studies can be combined for risk assessment and, as if that were not enough, a set of rules for actually bringing about such a synthesis. I must confess that I feel quite inadequate to this task. I do, however, have opinions on the appropriate approaches to combining epidemiological studies for risk assessment. One of the strongest held of these opinions is that each case must be treated on its own merits, and that canned recipes for combining studies are doomed to failure.

Much has recently been written on meta-analysis in epidemiology (Greenland, 1987; Fleiss and Gross, 1991; Dickersin and Berlin, 1992; MacClure, 1993). The problems faced by the would be meta-analyst can be summed up in a word: heterogeneity. Whether it is heterogeneity in the probability of publication (publication bias), in the quality of studies, in the measures of exposure and response used, or in the control of confounders, the analyst has been warned in many recent publications to guard against it. In the face of such heterogeneity and oftentimes insufficient data even to detect it, I am firmly of the opinion that an analytic approach, which treats meta-analysis as a 'study of studies' (Greenland, 1994) is vastly preferable to a synthetic approach, which attempts to arrive at a single estimate of risk derived from the studies considered (Greenland, 1994). However, the two approaches are not mutually exclusive. In many cases, after a careful review of the various studies, it may indeed be possible to select a subset that satisfies some predetermined criteria of excellence, and arrive at a consensus estimate of risk if it appears reasonable to do so, i.e., if there is no evidence of heterogeneity among the estimates of risk from the different studies. In practice, it may be difficult to rule out heterogeneity. Standard statistical tests for homogeneity of effects readily allow the rejection of homogeneity. The acceptance of homogeneity is not so simple. I am skeptical of formal criteria that suggest the acceptance of homogeneity if the p-value associated

Address for correspondence: Suresh Moolgavkar MD, PhD, Program in Biostatistics, Fred Hutchinson Cancer Research Center, 1124 Columbia Street, MP-665, Seattle, WA 98104, USA. Tel.: +1-206-667-4273. Fax: +1-206-667-7004.

with a statistical test for homogeneity crosses some predetermined threshold. If heterogeneity is detected, then I believe that every effort should be made to understand the sources of the heterogeneity. The use of random effects models to combine obviously disparate results is to be decried.

Combination of studies for risk assessment presents special problems. Risk assessment is part Science and part Black Magic. The risk assessor is almost always in the unenviable position of extrapolating risk down to levels where direct observation is impossible. For example, in the United States, the risk assessor is required to determine that dose of a putative environmental carcinogen which will lead to an increase in the lifetime probability of cancer of one in a million. Often he is required to perform this exercise even before it is determined that the agent in question is a human carcinogen. This is, of course, quite appropriate because the sole purpose of risk assessment is the protection of the public health. Thus, I believe that the risk assessor should be given some latitude to combine risk estimates from studies that appear to be discrepant. A specific example discussed below will make my point a little clearer, I hope.

I can think of at least four distinct situations in which one might want to combine evidence from different epidemiological studies for risk assessment.

1. To classify an agent as a human carcinogen. For example, both the International Agency for Research on Cancer (IARC) and the United States Environmental Protection Agency (USEPA) require "sufficient" epidemiological evidence of carcinogenicity before an agent is classified as a known human carcinogen. In this case I believe that the most stringent criteria should be applied in carrying out any kind of meta-analysis. Careful consideration should be given to the quality of individual studies and to the consistency of results from study to study. In short, the basic principles of meta-analysis summarized above, and discussed at length in recent publications, should be adhered to. An example of such a meta-analysis is provided by the recent EPA review of Dioxin. Epidemiological evidence of the carcinogenicity of Dioxin was evaluated from occupational cohort studies, case-control studies of soft tissue sarcomas and lymphomas, and from studies of populations exposed to Dioxin because of industrial accidents or poisoning of food. I do not intend to discuss this kind of meta-analysis further because it has already received much attention in the scientific literature.

2. Sometimes adequate, or even compelling, human evidence is available that an agent poses a risk to human health at high doses, but the effects at low exposures are not well understood. Oftentimes low-level exposures to such agents are ubiquitous and control measures may impose a large economic burden on society. Examples of such agents are radon and air pollution. However, these agents pose different challenges to the risk assessor. With air pollution, exposures are difficult, if not impossible, to measure on an individual level. Recently, there have been numerous reports, in the literature, of an increase in daily mortality associated with increase in measures of air pollution in various U.S. cities. These reports have been based on ecological studies. Particular attention has focused on the total suspended particulates (TSP) and more specifically on the PM_{10} (particulate matter

less than 10 μm in diameter) fraction. I believe that not enough attention has been paid to possible confounding factors and data combined (i.e., a "meta-analysis" performed) without proper consideration of whether such procedures were warranted. I will discuss some of these issues below.

3. In the case of radon, although individual exposures are difficult to measure, numerous cohort and case-control studies of radon and lung cancer are now available. The cohort studies have been conducted among underground miners who were exposed to relatively high levels of radon. The information on smoking ranges from being adequate to nonexistent in the various cohorts. More recently, case-control studies of lung cancer and residential radon exposure have been undertaken. The challenge is to construct a dose-response curve using all the information from the cohort and case-control studies.

4. As with most agents for which risk assessments are required, little direct human evidence of adverse health effects is available. Sometimes risk assessments are required for closely related agents, and some information may be available for only one, or a few, of a group of agents. For example, the polycyclic aromatic hydrocarbons (PAHs) are a group of organic compounds that have been shown to be carcinogenic in experimental systems and a few epidemiologic studies. However, the carcinogenic potencies of the different PAHs are different. Similarly, a number of polychlorinated biphenyls (PCBs) are strong tumor promoters and are considered to have dioxin like effects on biological systems. Typically, human exposure occurs, not to single compounds, but to mixtures of these compounds. Risk assessment is then sometimes based on the concept of toxicity equivalents, i.e., an easily measured biological end-point is used as a surrogate measure of carcinogenic potency. For example, with the dioxin-like PCBs, a toxicity equivalency factor (TEF) is estimated based on the efficiency, relative to dioxin, with which the agents induce the cytochrome p-450s. The carcinogenic potency of a mixture is then assumed to be directly proportional to the total TEF of the mixture. When some human data are available, a Bayesian approach originally proposed by DuMouchel and Harris (1983) can be used instead. I will illustrate by means of an example below.

Air pollution and daily mortality

A number of papers have recently reported an association between particulate air pollution and daily mortality in various metropolitan areas in the United States (e.g., Schwartz and Dockery, 1992a, 1992b). These publications treat daily mortality over the period of study as a time series, and use Poisson regression to estimate the effects of the covariates of interest on daily mortality. With few exceptions (Moolgavkar et al., 1995), these investigations have not performed the analyses separately by season. Separate analysis by season appears to be reasonable on a priori grounds. For example, one would expect the effects of weather to be different in summer and winter, with high temperatures contributing to mortality in the summer and cold temperatures contributing to mortality in the winter. Moreover, even if seasons are pulled out and analyzed separately, it is not clear that the same season from different years should be analyzed together. Thus, one might expect the severity of respiratory infections in winter, which depends upon the strain of virus making the rounds in any particular year, to interact with pollution in its effect on mortality. Further, a change in the demographics of the population over the period of study could also affect the estimates of the coefficients associated with air pollution, with a younger population expected to be less susceptible to the effects of air pollution than an older one. For these reasons I believe that the effects of air pollution on daily mortality should be investigated separately for each season and each year. If there is evidence of heterogeneity of results, then the reasons for such heterogeneity should be sought. If, on the other hand, there is little evidence of heterogeneity, then the estimates may be summarized into a single estimate.

I would like to discuss briefly an analysis of daily mortality in Philadelphia between 1973 and 1988. This was an analysis conducted in collaboration with Georg Luebeck, Elizabeth Anderson and Thomas Hall. I report here the results for the winter season, which was defined as comprising the months of December, January and February. Daily mortality was analyzed using the method of Poisson regression. The regression model included an intercept term, a term for the effect of sulfur dioxide and a term for the effect of total suspended particulates (TSP). In addition, temperature was discretized into quintiles and entered into the regression as a discrete covariate. After fitting the model there was no evidence of autocorrelation among the residuals, thus we adjusted the standard errors of the estimates only for overdispersion using standard techniques (McCullagh and Nelder, 1989).

The results of analyzing the data year by year are shown in Fig. 1. Figure 1 shows the estimated relative risks (and their 95% confidence intervals) associated with exposure to TSP and sulfur dioxide (top two panels) and with the lowest quintile of temperature (lowest panel). The figure suggests heterogeneity of effects from year to year, with the estimates for TSP appearing to be scattered randomly above and below relative risk 1, and the estimates for sulfur dioxide mainly above relative risk 1. Figure 2 shows the results of analyzing the entire 16 years after pooling the date, with common pollution and temperature coefficients for all years. As expected, the confidence intervals about the estimates are much tighter. Is such a summarization justified? Tests of heterogeneity indicate that single pollution coefficients for all years describe the data just as well as separate pollution coefficients for each year. Thus, the test for heterogeneity of pollution effects is highly nonsignificant (difference in deviances (after adjustment for overdispersion) = 33.1 on 30 degrees of freedom, p = 0.32). Similarly, the test for heterogeneity of effects of the lowest temperature quintile is highly nonsignificant. There is, thus, little evidence of heterogeneity in the effects of the pollution or temperature variables, and the summary representation seen in Fig. 2 is probably reasonable. Analyses of the other seasons, not shown here, lead to similar conclusions.

Figure 2 shows that both TSP and sulfur dioxide are significantly associated with mortality when each of them is considered separately in the regression model

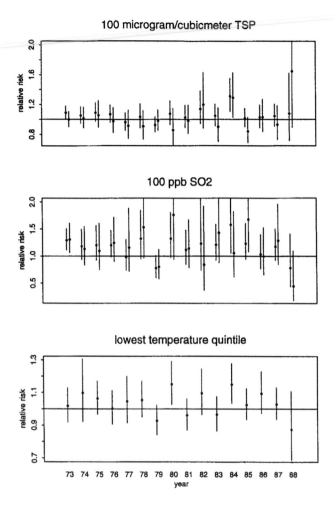

Fig. 1. Results of Poisson regression analysis of daily mortality in Philadelphia during winter. Each winter season beginning with the season of 1973, defined as December 1973, January and February 1974, and with the season of 1988, defined as December 1988, were analyzed separately. With the exception of the season of 1988, all other winters consisted of 3 months. No data were available after December 1988. For each season, the top panel shows the relative risks, together with their 95% confidence intervals, associated with exposure to 100 μg/m³ of TSP. The left member of each pair of vertical lines represents the relative risk estimated when TSP alone (together with quintiles of temperature and an intercept term) was included in the regression. The right member of the pair represents the relative risk associated with TSP when both TSP and sulfur dioxide were included in the model (in addition to the quintiles of temperature and the intercept term). The middle panel represents the relative risks and 95% confidence intervals associated with exposure to 100 parts per billion of sulfur dioxide. The interpretation of each pair of vertical lines is as given above, with the first line representing the risk associated with sulfur dioxide alone in the regression model, and the second the risk associated with sulfur dioxide with both TSP and sulfur dioxide in the regression model. The bottom panel represents the risk associated with the lowest quintile of temperature with TSP, sulfur dioxide and an intercept term included in the regression model in addition to the quintiles of temperature.

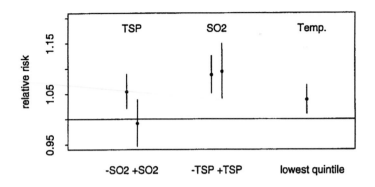

Fig. 2. Summary estimates of the relative risks and 95% confidence intervals associated with 100 μg/m³ of TSP, 100 ppb sulfur dioxide, and the lowest quintile of temperature. For TSP and sulfur dioxide the pair of vertical lines are to be interpreted as explained in the legend to Fig. 1. The TSP and sulfur dioxide relative risks were estimated from a regression model that assumed common effects of these pollutants in all 16 winters but different effects of temperature and different intercepts in the 16 winters. This model cannot be rejected when tested against the hierarchical model that postulates different pollution effects in each of the years, i.e., the model whose results are shown in Fig. 1. The temperature effect was estimated from a model that assumes the same temperature effect in all the 16 winters, but different pollution effects and intercepts. This model is strongly rejected by the likelihood ratio test when tested against the model of Fig. 1.

(together with quintiles of temperature). However, when both pollution covariates are included in the model (together with quintiles of temperature), the effect of TSP is greatly attenuated and the relative risk is estimated to be somewhat below 1, whereas the estimate of the sulfur dioxide coefficient remains virtually unchanged and remains highly statistically significant. This finding stands in contrast to recent reports of the relative importance of TSP and sulfur dioxide as determinants of daily mortality (Schwartz and Dockery, 1992b).

Radon and lung cancer

Studies in cohorts of underground miners, who are exposed to high levels of radon, leave little doubt that radon is a human carcinogen. Since exposure to radon is ubiquitous, there is concern that the typically low levels of radon exposure in homes may be causing some fraction of lung cancers in the general population. The miners' studies show that the relative risk associated with joint exposure to radon and cigarette smoke is somewhere between additive and multiplicative. There are now several case-control studies that have attempted directly to address the question of the risk posed by exposure to radon in homes. Taken together, these studies are inconclusive regarding the role of low exposures to radon in lung cancer. For a thoughtful discussion of the interpretation of these studies I refer the reader to a recent commentary by Lubin (1994). Figure 3, taken from that commentary, shows

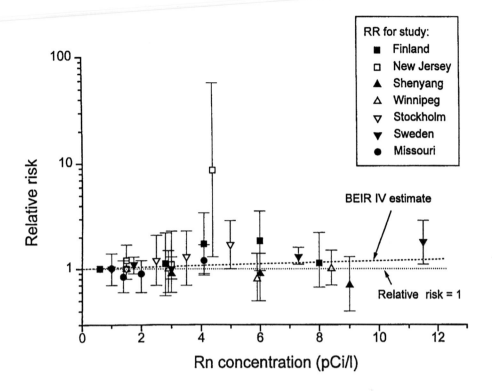

Fig. 3. Reproduced with permission from Lubin (1994). Relative risks (RR) for lung cancer by picocuries per liter (pCi/l) for the seven case-control studies of residential radon (Rn) exposure. Also shown are a plot of predicted relative risk for residential exposure from the age of 35–65 years using the model of the Committee on the Biological Effects of Ionizing Radiations (BEIR IV) adjusted to 1 pCi/liter as the referent exposure and a plot of relative risk of 1.0.

the relative risks obtained from seven case-control studies together with the dose-response curve constructed from the BEIR IV report. This dose-response curve is based on the miners' data. To me it appears as if there is remarkably good agreement among these studies and, for the purposes of risk assessment, I would be prepared to accept the estimates of risk predicted by the dose-response curve of the BEIR IV report. It must be remembered, however, that the BEIR IV dose-response curve is based on the assumption that there is no threshold for the effect of radon. So the question: is radon at levels present in homes a human carcinogen? remains an open one. Indeed, if meta-analysis is to be used to address that question, then the stringent criteria outlined above under item 1 must be observed before studies are combined. This could be problematic because the case-control studies are quite heterogeneous as Lubin points out in his commentary.

Without getting into the question of whether or not there is a threshold exposure below which radon is not a carcinogen, I will describe briefly an approach that can be used to combine dose-response curves from cohort and case-control studies of cancer. I assume here that the raw data are available from all the studies. If the studies can be considered to be independent, then the total likelihood function for all the studies is simply the product of likelihood functions from each of the studies. This likelihood can be maximized to yield estimates of parameters and statistical tests, based on the likelihood ratio principle, can be used to test for heterogeneity of the parameters from study to study.

Suppose now that we have a parametric hazard function for the end-point of interest. In the case we are considering here, this end-point is lung cancer. The parametric hazard function could be derived, for example, from the multistage model (Armitage and Doll, 1954) or the two-stage clonal expansion model of carcinogenesis (Moolgavkar et al., 1993). Let us denote this hazard function by $h(t \mid \beta, x)$, where t denotes age, x is a vector of covariates of interest and β a vector of parameters to be estimated. The vector x includes d, the exposure rate of the agent of interest, as one of its entries. Thus, in the case of radon, d would be the rate of exposure to radon. Other entries of x would be other covariates of interest, for example exposure to cigarette smoke measured in number of cigarettes smoked per day. The exposure rates can vary with time and age. Henceforth, for convenience, I will omit β from all expressions. Let $P(t \mid x)$ and $f(t \mid x)$ denote, respectively, the probability and the density functions associated with the hazard function h.

For cohort studies, the likelihood function is now easy to compute. If information is available on an individual basis in the cohort, i.e., if individual level covariate and failure (age of development of lung cancer) information are available, then the likelihood is constructed as follows. The likelihood contribution for an individual who develops lung cancer at age t is $f(t \mid x)$, where x is the vector of covariates for the individual including the pattern of exposure to radon and to cigarette smoke (if this information is available). An individual who dies of causes other than lung cancer, is lost to follow-up, or is alive at the end of the study is considered to be censored for the purposes of statistical analysis. The likelihood contribution for such an individual is $S(t \mid x)$, where S is the survivor function given by $S(t \mid x) = 1 - P(t \mid x)$.

If information in the cohort is not available on an individual level but only on subgroups as for example in the British doctors' cohort in which information is cross-tabulated by 5-year age groups and the number of cigarettes smoked per day in multiples of five, then the likelihood construction proceeds as follows. The number of lung cancer deaths in age group i and smoking level j is assumed to follow a Poisson distribution with mean $N_{ij}h(t \mid x_j)$, where N_{ij} represents the person-years at risk and x_j is the average of the covariates in that cell. Assuming that the number of events in any cell is independent of the number in any other cell, the full likelihood is the product of the individual Poisson likelihood contributions from each of the age-smoking categories.

The construction of the likelihood for case-control studies is somewhat more involved. I consider two cases separately.

Matched case-control study

When case by case matching is used, the construction of the likelihood is relatively simple. One view of an age-matched case-control study is as follows. Cases and controls are viewed as being drawn from a single cohort which is being followed forward in time. As individuals fail, controls are chosen randomly from among those in the risk set at that time (age). This view of a matched case-control study as a synthetic case-control or a case-control within a cohort study leads to the following likelihood contribution from each matched set. Suppose there are M matched sets, $m = 1, 2, \cdots, M$, with N_i controls associated with case i.

Then the likelihood contribution made by matched set i is:

$$L_i = \frac{h(t_i | x_0)}{\sum\limits_{j=0}^{N_i} h(t_i | x_j)},$$

where $h(t_i | x_0)$ is the hazard function for the ith case at the time of failure (t_i), and the sum in the denominator is taken over the case and all controls in risk set i. Note that in this formulation the hazard function for the controls is computed at time t_i which is the time (age) of failure of the case. Of course, in case-control studies such precise matching is impossible, as some controls are younger and other controls are older than the case. However, there are usually predetermined matching criteria, i.e., controls will be chosen only if their ages are within a certain age window (defined by the age of the case). To take account of this, it may be advisable to replace the hazard functions h above by the corresponding (conditional) probabilities of failure in the interval defined by the lower boundary of the age window and the age at which the case or control was sampled (conditional on failure not having occurred prior to the lower boundary of the age window). That is, the continuous hazard function h is replaced by a discrete version.

Stratified case-control study

Frequently in case-control studies, controls are not individually matched to cases. Instead "frequency" matching on confounding variables of interest is employed leading to a stratified study. Let us assume that strata are defined by values of a vector of matching variables, z. Assume further that there are S such strata indexed by $s = 1, 2, \cdots, S$, and that θ_{0s} is the sampling frequency of the cases in stratum s, i.e., the probability of sampling a case satisfying the criteria defining stratum s. Similarly, let θ_{1s} be the sampling frequency of controls. Typically, θ_{0s} is close to 1, whereas θ_{1s} is small. Suppose that in stratum s exactly m cases and n controls are sampled and $x_1, x_2, \cdots, x_m$ are the covariate vectors associated with the cases and $x_{m+1}, \cdots, x_{m+n}$ are the covariate vectors associated with the controls. Suppose that all failures occurred simultaneously at time t_s, then give n that the sample in stratum s consists of individuals with $m + n$ risk vectors $x_1, x_2, \cdots, x_m, \cdots, x_{m+n}$, the probability that the first m such vectors actually correspond to the cases is given by Prentice and Breslow (1978).

$$L_s = \theta_{1s}^m \theta_{0s}^n \prod_{j=1}^m h(t_s|x_j) \Big/ \sum_{l \in R(m,n)} \{ \theta_{1s}^m \theta_{0s}^n \prod_{j=1}^m h(t_s|x_{lj}) \}$$

$$= \prod_{j=1}^m h(t_s|x_j) \Big/ \sum_{l \in R(m,n)} \{ \prod_{j=1}^m h(t_s|x_{lj}) \}$$

where $R(m,n)$ is the set of all subsets of size m from $\{1, \cdots, m+n\}$. L_s is the likelihood contribution from stratum s and the total likelihood is, of course, the product of likelihood contributions from each of the strata.

As in the matched case-control situation described above, it may be advisable to replace h by a discretized version of h. More precisely, suppose the lower time (age) boundary of stratum s is defined by (t_{s-1}). Define $\tilde{h}(t_i \mid x_i) = \{$Prob that individual with covariates x_i fails in (t_{s-1}, t_i), conditional on his not having failed prior to $t_{s-1}\}$.

If the strata are large, then the likelihood given above presents computational problems because of the necessity of adding up $R(m,n)$ terms in the denominators of the stratum specific likelihood terms. Approximations suggested by Peto (1972) and Efron (1977) can then be used.

Another approach to analyzing stratified case-control data is to utilize the notion of the case-cohort design (Prentice, 1986). Suppose, as above, that there are exactly m cases and n controls in stratum s with covariates $x_1, \cdots, x_{m+n}$. Let $t_1, t_2, \cdots, t_m$ be the time (age) of failure of the m cases, and assume without loss of generality that $t_1 < t_2 < \cdots < t_m$ (if there are ties, they may be broken arbitrarily). Then for the ith case, let C_i be the set of controls whose ages are greater than or equal to t_i. Define the ith risk set in stratum s by $R_i = \{i^{th}$ case$\} \ U \ C_i$. The contribution to the likelihood made by R_i is:

$$\frac{h(t_i|x_i)}{\sum_{j \in C_i} h(t_i|x_j)}$$

where $h(t_i \mid x_j)$ is the hazard function at time t_i for the jth control in C_i. The likelihood contribution made by stratum s is the product of contribution over all risk sets and the total likelihood is the product of contributions made by each of the strata. The likelihood constructed in this fashion is a pseudo likelihood. The variance computation is known to be tricky and will need to be investigated.

Finally, if the sampling fractions θ_{0s} and θ_{1s} are known, or can be estimated, yet another approach to the analysis is possible. Let $h(t_i \mid x_i)$ be, as above, the discretized versions of the hazard function. By Bayes' theorem, the probability of failing in interval (t_{s-1}, t_i) conditional on covariates x and on being *sampled* and not having failed before t_{s-1}, is given by:

$$\tilde{P}(t_i|x_i) = \frac{\theta_{0s}\tilde{h}(t_i|x_i)}{\theta_{1s}(1-\tilde{h}(t_i|x_i)) + \theta_{0s}\tilde{h}(t_i|x_i)}.$$

Then, each case in stratum s will make contribution $\tilde{P}$ to the likelihood and each control will contribute $1 - \tilde{P}$. The total likelihood will, of course, be the product of such terms over all strata.

Because the hazard function used in the construction of the above likelihoods for case-control data is not of the proportional hazards form, the background hazard rate does not drop out of the expressions for the likelihood. This implies, in particular, that one should be able to obtain estimates of the background hazard rates from the case-control data. But, of course, it is well known that rates cannot be estimated from case-control data. One practical consequence of this is that the estimates of parameters obtained from an analysis of case-control data alone are likely to be highly unstable. Some external estimates of background rates are required. If the cohort study is large enough, then the background rates could be estimated from it. This procedure, however, requires the rather large assumption that the background rates in all the populations in which the case-control studies were conducted are similar and close to the background rates in the cohort studies.

The approach to combining case-control and cohort studies that I have described here will work only if the raw data are available. Various functional forms for the dose-response function for both radon exposure and cigarette smoking can be tried, and standard statistical tests based on the likelihood principle can be used to test for equality of parameters. For an example which uses this approach of a simultaneous analysis of the Colorado Plateau miners' data and the British doctors' data, see the recent publication by Moolgavkar et al. (1993).

A Bayesian approach when the data are sparse

This section is based on the work of DuMouchel and Harris (1983). They proposed a Bayesian approach for interspecies extrapolation of dose-response functions. However, the method can be used when the risk associated with exposure to an agent has to be estimated without direct information in the population of interest. Information, however, is available on the agent in other populations and information on closely related agents may be available in the population of interest. A summarized example from the BEIR IV report illustrates the basic principles of this approach. The principal goal of the analysis was to estimate the risk of bone cancer in humans following exposure to two isotopes of Plutonium, ^{238}Pu and ^{239}Pu. Plutonium is an α-emitter and no human information on these isotopes of Plutonium was available. Human information was available, however, on two isotopes of Radium, ^{236}Ra and ^{228}Ra, which are also α-emitters. The available information is summarized in Table 1, which is modified from the BEIR IV report.

The first step in using the method proposed by DuMouchel and Harris is to

Table 1. Summary of available data.

Biological system	Isotope			
	^{226}Ra	^{228}Ra	^{238}Pu	^{239}Pu
Human	+	+	−	−
Beagle dog (injection)	+	+	−	+
Beagle dog (inhalation)	−	−	+	−
Rat	−	−	+	+

Note: + indicates that data are available in this cell; − indicates no available data.

reanalyze each one of the data sets in the same way. In each data set, there was sufficient information only for a rather rudimentary analysis. A simple Poisson model was fit by maximum likelihood to each of the data sets. Let N be the number of individuals in a given dose-group, n the number of individuals who died of bone cancer, T the total person-days of exposure, and D the sum of the cumulative doses in rads up to death, or time of last contact of each individual in the dose group. The assumption then was that n has a Poisson distribution with mean $E(n) = \lambda D(1 - \tau N/T)$, where λ is an estimate of the potency (slope of the dose-response curve) and τ is the latent period.

Now let y_{ij} be the estimated ln (λ_{ij}) in the ith row and j^{th} column of Table 1, and assume that y_{ij} is normally distributed conditional on the true log slope, θ_{ij}, so that $y_{ij} \mid \theta_{ij} \sim N(\theta_{ij}, c_{ij}^2)$. The θ in turn have normal prior distributions, so that $\theta_{ij} \mid (\alpha, \gamma, \sigma) \sim N(\alpha_i + \alpha_i, \gamma_i, \sigma)$. Thus α_i is a measure of the sensitivity of the ith biological system to the average isotope, and γ_j is a measure of the average potency of the jth isotope across the biological systems. Finally, the parameters α_i, γ_j and σ have prior distributions that are specified on the basis of biological information. For details, see annex 7a in the BEIR IV report. With the model specified in this way, the empty cells in Table 1 can be filled in. Based on such an analysis, the BEIR IV report concludes that the risk of bone cancer death is about 300 per million person rad of internally deposited plutonium, with the 95% confidence interval extending from 80–1100 bone cancer deaths.

Although the analysis described here combines information from animal and human studies, similar methods can be applied to studies of similar, but not identical, agents in different human populations.

Concluding remarks

I have argued here, principally by example, that the goals of risk assessment do not necessarily coincide with those of sound epidemiologic analysis. Consequently, the risk assessor must be given considerable leeway in the use of meta-analytic techniques. This is not to say that all considerations of the quality of individual studies used in the meta-analysis should be jettisoned. The risk assessor simply has to use different criteria from the epidemiologist. It could be argued that the levels of risk that the risk assessor is required to estimate are unreasonable and that regulation should be based on more realistic assessments of risk. For example, I do not believe that we will ever be in a position to predict accurately the dose of an agent that increases lifetime cancer risk by 1 in a million. But this is missing the point.No matter what regulatory criteria are used, the risk assessor, more often than not, is going to be faced with the problem of inadequate data. When data are actually available in human populations at the low levels of exposure where regulation is to take place, then the same stringent criteria that have been developed for epidemiologic studies should be applied. Air pollution is a case in point.

As I have pointed out earlier, the main concern of the meta-analyst is with heterogeneity. But this is a problem that every epidemiologic study faces. Even with single studies, the epidemiologist is faced with the issues of whether or not risks are constant from stratum to stratum (no effect modification), and, if they are deemed to be constant, whether the strata can be collapsed (no confounding by the stratifying variables). Every epidemiologic study begins with the implicit belief that, at least for the purposes of the study, populations can be subdivided into homogeneous subgroups. Later information may reveal that, in fact, the assumptions of homogeneity were unjustified. For instance, it is now becoming increasingly clear that inter-individual variations in metabolic phenotype, as exemplified by debrisoquine metabolism and the rate of metabolism of aromatic amines (acetylator phenotype), greatly influence the risk associated with exposure to carcinogenic agents. A couple of studies have shown approximately 5-fold increases in lung cancer inextensive metabolizers of debrisoquine (Ayesh et al., 1984; Caporaso et al., 1990). Slow acetylators are at increased risk of bladder cancer (Mommsen et al., 1985). Stratification on these variables is important in future studies.

The remarks made here are not meant to trivialize the difficulties faced by meta-analysis, but to point out that, without some assumptions of homogeneity, epidemiologic studies would not be possible. While every attempt should be made to follow the sound principles of meta-analysis enunciated in recent papers, ultimately how these principles are put into practice will depend on the particular circumstances under which the analysis is undertaken. Finally, there will always be a strong subjective component to meta-analysis, particularly meta-analysis undertaken for the purposes of risk assessment.

Acknowledgements

Research supported in part by grants from NCI and DOE.

References

Armitage P and Doll R. The age distribution of cancer and a multistage theory of carcinogenesis. Br J Cancer 1954;8:1–12.

Ayesh R, Idle JR, Ritchie JC and Crothers MJ. Metabolic oxidation phenotypes as markers for susceptibility to lung cancer. Nature 1984;312(5990):169–170.

BEIR IV. Health Risks of Radon and Other Internally Deposited Alpha-Emitters. Washington, D.C.: National Academy Press, 1988.

Caporaso NE, Tucker MA, Hoover RN, Hayes RB, Pickle LW, Issaq HJ, Muschik GM, Green-Gallo L, Buivys D, Aisner S et al. Lung cancer and the debrisoquine metabolic phenotype. J Natl Cancer Inst 1990;82(15):1264–1272.

Dickersin K and Berlin JA. Meta-analysis: state-of-the-science. Epidemiol Rev 1992;14:154–176.

DuMouchel WH and Harris JE. Bayes methods for combining the results of cancer studies in humans and other species. J Am Stat Assoc 1983;78(382):293–315.

Efron B. The efficiency of Cox's likelihood for censored data. J Am Stat Assoc 1977;72:557–565.

Fleiss JL and Gross AJ. Meta-analysis in epidemiology, with special reference to studies of the association between exposure to environmental tobacco smoke and lung cancer: a critique. J Clin Epidemiol 1991;44(2):127–139.

Greenland S. Quantitative methods in the review of epidemiologic literature. Epidemiol Rev 1987;9:1–30.

Greenland S. Invited Commentary: A critical look at some popular meta-analytic methods. Am J Epidemiol 1994;140(3):290–296.

Lubin JH. Invited commentary: Lung cancer and exposure to residential radon. Am J Epidemiol 1994; 140(4):323–332.

Maclure M. Demonstration of deductive meta-analysis: ethanol intake and risk of myocardial infarction. Epidemiol Rev 1993;15(2):328–351.

McCullagh P and Nelder JA. Generalized Linear Models. 2nd edn. New York: Chapman and Hall, 1989.

Mommsen S, Barfod NM and Aagaard J. N-acetyltransferase phenotypes in the urinary bladder carcinogenesis of a low-risk population. Carcinogenesis 1985;6(2):199–201.

Moolgavkar SH, Luebeck EG, Hall TA and Anderson EL. Particulate air pollution, sulfur dioxide, and daily mortality: A reanalysis of the Steubenville data. Inhalation Toxicol 1995;7:35–44.

Moolgavkar SH, Luebeck EG, Krewski D and Zielinski JM. Radon, cigarette smoke, and lung cancer: a reanalysis of the Colorado Plateau uranium miners' data. Epidemiology 1993;4(3):204–217.

Peto R. Contribution to the discussion of paper by D.R. Cox. J Roy Stat Soc 1972;34(B):205–207.

Prentice RL. A case-cohort design for epidemiologic cohort studies and disease prevention trials. Biometrika 1986;73:1–11.

Prentice RL and Breslow N. Retrospective studies and failure time models. Biometrika 1978;65:153–158.

Schwartz J and Dockery DW. Particulate air pollution and daily mortality in Steubenville, Ohio. Am J Epidemiol 1992a;135(1):12–25.

Schwartz J and Dockery DW. Increased mortality in Philadelphia associated with daily air pollution concentrations. Am Rev Resp Dis 1992b;145:600–604.

©1995 Elsevier Science B.V. All rights reserved.
The Role of Epidemiology in Regulatory Risk Assessment
J.D. Graham, editor.

Principles for guidelines on when and how to combine results from multiple epidemiologic studies in risk assessment

Malcolm Maclure

ScD Associate Professor, Epidemiology Department, Harvard School of Public Health, Boston Massachusetts, and Manager, Statistical Analysis and Surveys, Research and Evaluation Branch, British Columbia Ministry of Health, Victoria, British Columbia, Canada

Key words: assessment, decision, dose-response, epidemiology, extrapolation, regulators, risk.

In this commentary, aimed at regulators and risk assessors, I address Prof Graham's question: What principles should guide the development of guidelines for using epidemiologic evidence in risk assessment? My original, but now secondary purpose, is to comment on the paper by Moolgavkar.

Moolgavkar's paper is a good academic paper, but illustrates the cultural gap between academic researchers and decision makers (Table 1). I recognize this gap because I have both an academic position but work on decision-oriented topics in a provincial health department. My commentary will attempt to bridge this gap.

Summary of Moolgavkar's paper

Moolgavkar is "against canned recipes", and says there are "no set rules for combining..." results. He says seldom is it possible for a meta-analyst to produce a summary estimate of excess risk, so risk assessors must be given more latitude than meta-analysts. He mentions four situations when one might want to combine results:
a. Hazard identification: yes or no. Does the agent have *any* health effect, however small? His advice is to refer to epidemiologists' papers on meta-analysis including mine (Maclure, 1993).
b. Extrapolation to low doses. He warns that too often too little attention is paid to confounders, such as controlling for SO_2 when looking at the relation of total suspended particulates in the air and excess mortality rates.

Address for correspondence: Malcom MacLure, Associate Professor of Epidemiology, Kresge 902, Havard School of Public Health, 667 Huntington Avenue, Boston, MA 02115, USA. Tel.: +1-617−432−1199. Fax: +1-617−566−7805.
Alternative address: Research and Evaluation Branch, Ministry of Health, 1515 Blanchard Street, Victoria, British Columbia, Canada V8W 3C8. Tel.: +1-604-952-2300. Fax: +1-604-952-2308.

Table 1.

The culture of academic researchers	The culture of decision makers
— Reluctant to generalize.	— Forced to generalize.
— Assumes audience can refer to literature.	— No time. Needs a snapshot summary of literature.
— Most interesting case is sophisticated analysis when you have lots of data.	— Most interesting case is when there is controversy. Often little data is available.
— No set rules. But there are ways *not* to do it.	— We do use rules already. Can't you improve them?
— Treat each case on its own merits.	— What characteristics are usually merits or demerits? Are there no patterns in these characteristics?
— A complicated answer is better if it is true, even if it is confusing.	— A correct result via obscure mathematics is worse than a nearly correct result via easy-to-understand mathematics.

c. Completing the dose-response curve using all data from cohort and case-control studies: The bulk of his paper is devoted to showing how to do this by computing the joint likelihood of all the data given various hypothesized hazard functions, and picking the result that maximizes this likelihood. However, he says raw data are required for this procedure.

d. Between-species and between-chemical extrapolation. He advises use of a Bayesian approach.

My chief criticism of Moolgavkar's paper is that, fine though it is as an academic paper, it does not address the concerns of decision makers. I will now show an alternative approach.

Rationale of our conference

Thorne Aucher explained that many legislators now want to attach to new environmental legislation, a requirement for "risk assessment that is objective and unbiased". I suggest the following interpretations:

"Objective" should be interpreted as *evidence-based, documented, and accessible rather than purely opinion-based or inaccessible.*

"Unbiased" should be interpreted as *conforming to procedures used by experts with no financial or personal preference for any particular result.*

Such a requirement and interpretation will create a demand for official definitions of evidence and official guidelines for procedures, which regulators can use for "assurance of quality of the process of risk assessment". If epidemiologists want such definitions and guidelines to be good, some of us must participate in creating them.

Recommended strategy: use reverse reasoning

A common sense approach to problem solving is to suppress prejudgment, look at the data, and then draw conclusions. Contrary to common sense, the opposite approach usually produces better results. It is often better to imagine alternative conclusions (to cultivate prejudgment) then find data that can help discriminate among these alternatives, and finally rank the conclusions according to how consistent they are with the data. Here I shall call this "reverse reasoning", because Professor Graham introduced the term "reverse guidance". It is reverse reasoning in the sense that it starts with conclusions. (A technical term for it is the hypothetico-deductive method.) I demonstrated this approach in my meta-analysis (Maclure, 1993) and it is explained in a paper on multivariate analysis (Maclure, 1990).

This approach was explicit in Moolgavkar's paper and implicit in Graham's paper. Moolgavkar advocates likelihood methods, Bayesian approaches, and meta-analyses that are explanatory rather than summative, all of which are based on reverse reasoning (Maclure, 1990). Graham favors risk assessment according to prior guidelines rather than rules developed for each case, and proposes that communication between epidemiologists and risk assessors should involve "reverse guidance" — risk assessors guiding epidemiologists.

Reverse guidance was not used in our conference. How might it have looked if it had been? Imagine if the conference had begun with a hypothetical set of guidelines drawn up by risk assessors, and the mission: please criticize and modify these draft guidelines. It would have been quite a different conference. Not all differences would have been improvements but, on average, I think the results would have been more usable by decision makers.

The criticism is often made that it is impossible for epidemiologists to agree on guidelines. This is a testable hypothesis. We should aim to produce guidelines and attempt to refute this criticism. We should use a method analogous to steps in a research study (see Table 2).

Regulator's needs

First, let us extend the reverse reasoning to its limit. Suppose the regulator complies with the legislation by commissioning an "objective, unbiased risk assessment". Let us now imagine a conversation when the risk assessor delivers an assessment to the regulator.

Table 2.

Steps in research	Steps for developing guidelines
— Translate biologic hypotheses into epidemiologic hypotheses.	— "Reverse Guidance": Risk assessors describe their approaches to epidemiologists, who then suggest alternatives.
— Define scope of the study.	— Agree on scope of guidelines.
— Collect data for testing hypothesis.	— Test guidelines in focus groups and by participant observation.
— Present results in standardized format.	— Document evidence and opinions for and against in an electronically accessible "paper trail".
— Discuss results for the educated lay readers.	— Discuss results in lay terms for use in public consultation.
— Track citations of the research paper.	— Monitor utilization of the guidelines.
— Design an experiment to test hypothesis more rigorously.	— Evaluate impact of guidelines comparing users with nonusers.

Regulator: "What guidelines did you use for your risk assessment?"
Risk assessor: "I used [one of the following]...
— my own judgement (no guidelines)
— the so-called "Explanatory Guidelines"
— the "Cross Design Synthesis" guidelines
— the so-called "Deductive Guidelines"
— all three, plus my own approach, and compared results."
Regulator: "What are the differences among these types of guidelines?"
Risk assessor: "Of course, there are proponents and critics of each."

Explanatory guidelines
Proponents: "Our goal should be to explain differences among results, not to combine results."
Critics: "This approach is indecisive; it passes the buck to regulators."

Cross-design synthesis guidelines
Proponents: "The goal should be a best summary of all results, which is what regulators need."
Critics: "This approach glosses over major potential explanations."

Deductive guidelines
Proponents: "The goal should be to test alternative decisions against evidence and

criticisms."
Critics: "This approach is contrary to common practice and complex."

This conversation is hypothetical. The three types of guidelines do not yet exist. They are my speculations, reflecting (so far) three different approaches to meta-analysis: explanatory (Greenland, 1994; Rubin, 1992), summative (Program evaluation and methodology division of the USA General Accounting Office, 1992), and deductive (Maclure, 1993).

Tactics

The strategy of reverse reasoning, outlined in Table 2, raises questions of tactics. Here are some suggestions:
a. *Reverse guidance.* The brainstorming should start with regulators informing risk assessors what they want, and then risk assessors explaining to epidemiologists how they would respond. Together they should develop a long list of interesting hypothetical guidelines.
b. *Scope.* I recommend that guidelines for scientific standards of criticisms should also be created. The need for this is evident from Dr. Feinstein's bombastic but nonquantitative critique presented at this conference which does not acknowledge the existence of quantitative solutions to the problems he says have not been addressed (Greenland, 1991). I am not the first to say Dr. Feinstein's approach to criticism does not need scientific standards (Savitz et al., 1990).
c. *Tests.* The list of hypothetical guidelines should be grouped and tested in focus groups, not only of professionals, but also nonprofessionals. All sets of guidelines should be accessible and intelligible to the general public.
   Given there are several different approaches to meta-analysis, attitudes towards guidelines will probably cluster into two or three schools of thoughts. It may be advisable to aim for a limited number of alternative sets of guidelines. This will enable specificity of guidelines to be achieved without excess rigidity.
d. *Publication.* Guidelines for risk assessors may face the same fate as clinical practice guidelines (CPGs) for health care. CPGs are much less effective than hoped, in part, because they often raise many more questions than they answer. A possible solution has been invented: "just-in-time knowledge" — publication of CPGs as evolving hypertext on the Internet's World Wide Web (Penn and Maclure, 1995). (A hypertext version of this paper can be found at "http://synapse.uah.alberta.ca/synapse/00000006.htm" which is an Internet World Wide Web address.) Each contentious phrase of the guidelines can be linked electronically, instantaneously to another document on any computer in the Internet, which can then be retrieved instantly with one key stroke. Thus evidence, supportive arguments, criticisms, counterarguments, and rebuttles can all be linked into one hypertext.
e. *Public access.* To make the hypertext guidelines accessible and intelligible to the

Table 3. Examples of possible guidelines for use of epidemiological data in risk assessment.

1. Ask investigators for intermediate analyses that were not publishable.
2. Use both risk ratio and risk difference to describe the excess risk.
3. Present a range of results and indicate what assumptions/procedures that the results are most sensitive to.
4. Use meta-analyses of evidence concerning hypothesized biases if available.
5. Hypotheses of residual confounding, selection bias, or misclassification bias should be expressed quantitatively as relative risk ratios, or risk difference changes.
6. Use "causal criteria" as a way of assessing unmeasured potential confounders and biases.
7. Adjust slope for measurement error only after 19 out of 20 epidemiologists say the association is probably causal.

public, they should deal with old arguments, even such ancient criticisms as "statistics are damn lies". Old arguments are new to many in the general public. Novices should be respected and given easy access to explanations of, and answers to, their concerns in their own language.

f. *Utilization and impact.* If the impossibility of guidelines is refuted, then the next criticisms to refute are that they are misused, ineffective, or harmful. Plans to test these hypotheses should be framed during the early phase of guideline use, otherwise a window of testability may be missed.

Do not use *quality-scores*[1]
Use *quality-component analysis*[2]

[1]It is common sense to give more weight to a good study and less to a poor study. Some *researchers*[A] tried doing this formally by assigning quality scores to studies. Their results led to the discovery that common sense was misleading.[B]*Critics disagree.*[C]

[A][Link to examples]

[B]For example, a study with two weaknesses both of which cause over-estimation would be treated as equally misleading as a study with two weaknesses that tend to cancel each other out. This is misleading.

[C][Link to critiques]

[2]This is an analysis that quantitatively explores various possible explanations for why the results of different studies differ. Is it mainly attributable to differences in study design? Are differences among results more related to differences among data collection methods? This approach has been discussed by *Greenland.*[A]

[A] [Link to Greenland's paper]

Fig. 1. Hypothetical guideline with hypertext links.

Examples

As a contribution to the brainstorming process, I offer some hypothetical guidelines (Table 3). I also show two examples of guidelines in hypertext format (Figs. 1 and 2).

Conclusion

In this commentary, I have used a little reverse reasoning. I started with the prediction that risk assessments will be increasingly mandated by legislation. Therefore, risk assessors will use whatever guidelines or checklists they can find. How will they deduce whether one set or another can stand up to evidence and criticism? No such guidelines have been systematically developed by critical peer review. Here I have illustrated how such guidelines can be developed.

Do not use the phrase *negative study*.[1] Use the phrases:
***Inconclusive study*,[2] or**
***Inverse result*[3] or,**
***Null result*[4]**

[1]List of examples

[2]If the 95% confidence intervals are wider than a factor of 3 and includes the null, refer to this as inconclusive because the results are consistent with both no effect and a *substantial effect*.[A] *Critics disagree*.[B]

   [A]A substantial effect is generally regarded as "more likely than not" to have caused the effect if exposed, i.e. a relative risk of 2.

   [B]Whether the null is just in or just out of the 95% confidence interval is another manifestation of the *fallacy* of significance testing. *Proponents disagree*.[ii]

      [i] It is still an improvement. "Inconclusive" is a rough description, not a decision to disregard the study.

      [ii] [Proponents' papers.]

[3]If the upper bound of 95% confidence interval < 1.

[4]Evidence in *favor* of *no* effect is difficult to produce. If a meta-analysis of randomized trials gave a relative risk between 0.95 and 1.05, with a 95% confidence interval of ± 0.05, most epidemiologists would agree to call this a null result.

Fig. 2. Hypothetical guideline with hypertext links.

References

Greenland S. A mathematical analysis of the "Epidemiologic necropsy". Annal Epidemiol 1991;1:551–558.

Greenland S. Invited commentary: a critical look at some popular meta-analytic methods. Am J Epidemiol 1994;140:290–296.

Maclure M. Demonstration of deductive meta-analysis: ethanol intake and risk of myocardial infarction. Epidemiol Rev 1993;15:328–351.

Maclure M. Multivariate refutation of etiologic hypotheses in nonexperimental epidemiology. Int J Epidemiol 1990;19:782–787.

Penn AMW, Maclure M. The synapse project: just-in-time knowledge. Ann R Coll Phys Surg Can 1995; (in press).

Program Evaluation and Methodology Division of United States General Accounting Office. Cross-design synthesis: a new strategy for medical effectiveness research. Washington DC, GAO/PEMD 1992;18.

Rubin DB. Meta-analysis: literature synthesis or effect-size surface estimation? J Educ Stat 1992;17:363–374.

Savitz DA, Greenland S, Stolley PD and Kelsey JL. Scientific standards of criticism: a reaction to Scientific standards in epidemiologic studies of the menace of daily life by A.R. Feinstein. Epidemiology 1990;1:78–83.

©1995 Elsevier Science B.V. All rights reserved.
The Role of Epidemiology in Regulatory Risk Assessment
J.D. Graham, editor.

Risk assessment, epidemiology, meta-analysis, and pooling

Earl Ford

Division of Nutrition, Centers for Disease Control and Prevention, Atlanta, Georgia, USA

Key words: assays, assessment, epidemiology, meta-analysis, pooling, risk, structure activity, toxicity.

Although more than 65,000 chemicals are estimated to be in commercial use in the United States, only about 10,000 have been tested for animal toxicity and less than 1,000 have been the subject of an epidemiologic study (Ladou, 1990; Griffith et al., 1993). Every year, the Environmental Protection Agency receives about 2,200–2,500 premanufacture notifications most of which are for new chemicals. Few of these chemicals have been subjected to rigorous evaluations concerning their safety to humans. Most certainly do not undergo the rigorous evaluation for safety that the pharmaceutical industry must conduct prior to receiving permission to market their drugs.

As evidence about the toxicity of a substance emerges, a risk assessment may be initiated. Risk assessment is generally presented as consisting of four main components: hazard identification, dose-response assessment, exposure assessment, and risk characterization (NRC, 1983). This process requires numerous sources of data from various disciplines. Data concerning the toxic potential of substances emanate largely from four lines of evidence: assays for mutagenicity and geno-toxicity, animal studies, structure-activity relationships, and epidemiologic studies.

The role of epidemiology in risk assessment

Since the end result of many risk assessments is the prediction of risk to humans from exposure, ideally one would like to have human data available. Risk assessors dealing with environmental exposures are unlikely to have the luxury of data from randomized clinical trials available to them. Therefore, epidemiologic studies, largely case-control and cohort studies, can provide important human data for a risk assessment. However, observational studies are subject to numerous methodologic difficulties.

Epidemiology can play an important role in two components of the risk assessment

---

Address for correspondence: Earl Ford, Radiation Studies Branch, National Center for Environmental Health, Centers for Disease Control and Prevention, 4770 Buford Highway, NE, Mailstop F35, Atlanta, GA 30341, USA. Tel.: +1-404-488-7040. Fax: +1-404-488-7044.

process: in hazard identification and in dose-response assessment. In hazard identification, the types of health effects from exposure are defined. Epidemiologic studies in addition to toxicologic studies and structure-activity relationships provide the relevant information. In dose-response assessment, data from epidemiologic studies or from animal studies define the quantitative relationship between exposure and health outcomes.

The role of meta-analysis and pooling in epidemiology and risk assessment

For many substances epidemiologic data are either lacking or sparse. However, sometimes a large body of epidemiologic data are available. For example, numerous studies have been conducted for radon, asbestos, formaldehyde, lead, polychlorinated biphenyls, metals, and environmental tobacco smoke. Because the risk assessor must define relevant health outcomes from an exposure and develop a best estimate of dose-response, some process is needed to summarize and combine the data or results of these studies.

Summarizing results from studies has a long tradition in science, especially in the form of the review article. Traditionally, most of these summaries have been narrative in format and have the tendency to be largely qualitative and somewhat subjective. However, the inadequacies of such reviews have been recognized, and as a result these studies have taken a more quantitative slant during the last two decades. Rosenthal, in a recent review, presents an example in which reviewers using meta-analysis to review seven papers were less likely to reject an association than was a group of reviewers who reviewed the same papers using classical techniques (Rosenthal, 1991).

Two major techniques in producing summary estimates from epidemiologic studies are pooling and meta-analysis. Pooling involves working with the primary data from individual studies by combining these into a database that can then be analyzed if the studies are sufficiently compatible. In meta-analysis, however, the analyst uses the end results of the analysis rather than the raw data. What distinguishes these from more traditional reviews and summaries is the quantitative approach to integrating data and results.

Although pooling may be a preferable approach in producing summary estimates, difficulties in obtaining data from the investigators of all studies may result in unsuccessful efforts. Pooling offers several advantages over meta-analysis. The availability of data leads to more flexibility in examining the data. Different models can be examined, common definitions and coding for health outcomes, exposures, confounders and effect modifiers can be developed, confounding, interaction, and effect modification can be more fully evaluated, and data anomalies can be investigated. Because of these advantages, results from pooled analyses are thought to be more valid. A good example of pooling is found in the radon literature where raw data from several mining cohorts were pooled to produce a pooled estimate of risk of lung cancer mortality from radon exposure (NRC, 1988). A recent article discusses various aspects of pooling methodology (Friedenreich, 1993).

The use of meta-analysis has exploded in epidemiology in recent years. In 1976, Glass introduced the term meta-analysis and defined it as "the statistical analysis of a large collection of analysis results from individual studies for the purpose of integrating the findings" (Glass, 1976). Meta-analysis can be useful in several ways. Because many studies have insufficient statistical power by themselves, meta-analysis can help improve the power of the combined studies if they are deemed to be combinable. Furthermore, meta-analysis may provide a better estimate of the effect size. Because studies in some instances yield inconsistent results, some have argued that meta-analysis has a role in smoothing out the data to come up with a single answer. This use of meta-analysis, however, is being increasingly criticized (Greenland, 1994). Instead, meta-analysis can provide a structured framework for sorting out the question of why studies may arrive at different conclusions. Also, meta-analysis can be a useful approach to illuminating inadequacies in the existing database and provide useful insights into future research needs (O'Rourke and Detsky, 1989). By demonstrating past inadequacies in studies, meta-analysis can also help to improve the quality of future studies. Finally, meta-analysis can increase the generalizability of the findings (Furberg and Morgan, 1987; Thompson and Pocock, 1991).

The use of meta-analysis is perhaps more straightforward with randomized clinical controlled trials than with observational studies because randomized clinical trials are generally acknowledged to be superior study designs. However, randomized clinical trials of most environmental exposures are not possible, and, therefore, much of the human evidence of risk, for risk assessment comes from epidemiologic studies. Because epidemiologic studies are not as free from biases as randomized clinical trials, meta-analysis of these studies is somewhat more problematic and requires more care (Spitzer, 1991; Fleiss and Gross, 1991).

How can meta-analysis and how will meta-analysis be used in risk assessment? Dr. Moolgavkar, in his interesting paper, provides insights into how meta-analysis can be used in risk assessment. He presents four situations in which meta-analysis would prove useful. Like other authors, he stresses the importance of looking for and pursuing the reasons for heterogeneity among studies. He proceeds to offer additional insights into methodology for combining dose-response curves from cohort and case-control studies and a method for extrapolating data from one population to another where few data may be available.

Meta-analysis and pooling can be a useful tools in two of the four steps in risk assessment: hazard identification and dose-response assessment. Because regulators and elected officials often desire a single risk estimate, there is considerable pressure to provide a central estimate. Meta-analysis can provide an approach to obtain such an estimate. However, Greenland cautions against the use of meta-analysis as a cookbook recipe for combining studies to provide a single estimate (Greenland, 1994). Rather, he views meta-analysis as a study of studies in which the investigator should approach each meta-analysis as a unique event and perform a thoughtful analysis of the studies.

Numerous articles and books have been written about the subject of meta-analysis. Some of the important concepts of meta-analysis include a diligent search of all applicable research, proper review of studies, decision framework for inclusion and exclusion of studies, study quality assessment, statistical techniques, and sensitivity analyses (L'Abbé et al., 1987; Sacks et al., 1987; Thacker, 1988). Jenicek has reviewed sources of bias to be avoided in a meta-analysis. These biases include the failure to find all relevant studies (retrieval bias, publication bias, conformity publication bias, search bias, reference bias, multiple publications bias, multiple used subjects bias), selection bias (inclusion criteria bias, selector bias), and bias in obtaining accurate data from selected studies (extractor bias, bias in scoring study quality, reporting bias, recording error) (Jenicek, 1989). Various references present information about the statistical techniques that are used in meta-analysis (Hedges and Olkin, 1985; Greenland, 1987; Laird and Mosteller, 1990; Greenland and Longnecker, 1992; Fleiss, 1993; Berlin et al., 1993; Pettiti, 1994). Reviews of elements of a good quality meta-analysis have also been published (L'Abbé et al., 1987; Sacks et al., 1987; Thacker, 1988).

Some cautions about the use of meta-analysis should be heeded. All too often meta-analysis is considered to be the definitive work on a topic. However, it should be recognized that a meta-analysis is only as good as the data and care that went into performing the analysis. There are clearly questions about meta-analysis, and especially meta-analysis of epidemiologic studies, that need to be answered. Spitzer, in a commentary on meta-analysis, lists a number of such questions. Controversial issues are how investigators set inclusion and exclusion criteria, the wisdom of using quality scores (Thompson and Pocock, 1991; Greenland, 1994), the conceptual framework to approaching meta-analysis (MacClure, 1993), and how to deal with heterogeneity of studies (Thompson and Pocock 1991; Greenland, 1994). Furthermore, what effect that meta-analysis may have on future research is also unclear.

Uncertainty analysis is becoming increasingly important in risk assessments. In the traditional epidemiologic literature, uncertainty analysis is largely synonymous with measurement error. For example, uncertainty analysis in the calculation of individual doses is an important issue in radiation epidemiology. In doing radiation dose reconstructions, an attempt is made to quantify sources of error and lack of knowledge in producing a dose probability distribution for each individual. The confidence intervals typically presented in the epidemiologic literature are solely based on sampling variation and do not include allowances for uncertainty. However, inclusion of uncertainty affects dose-response parameters and leads to broader uncertainty confidence intervals also known as credibility intervals (NIH, 1985).

A recent report from the Office of Technology Assessment identifies at least 12 federal agencies, institutes, and centers as employing risk assessment. Therefore, it is likely that these agencies will also employ meta-analysis or pooled analysis to provide data needed to complete risk assessments. However, the role of these techniques was summarized in one small paragraph. Given the numerous government organizations that will likely use meta-analysis, the question can be posed whether some effort should be made to develop a set of guidelines for performing meta-analysis to assure some degree of uniformity.

In summary, meta-analysis and pooling are useful tools in the process of risk assessment in providing summary estimates of dose-response and in the critical evaluation of human studies when these are available. Unfortunately, epidemiologic data are too often absent or insufficient. Nicholson summarizes some of the data with regard to animal and human studies of the carcinogenic potential of toxic substances (Nicholson, 1992). Of 400 chemicals with sufficient or limited data animal carcinogenicity that were reviewed by the International Agency for Research on Cancer, only 20 substances had sufficient human data. Therefore, it is of paramount importance to generate the necessary data. In developing such studies, the future role of meta-analysis should be kept in mind. Study designs and protocols should be kept as compatible as possible to facilitate subsequent pooled analyses or meta-analyses. Furthermore, meta-analyses may need to be repeated and updated as newer information becomes available or the methodology of meta-analysis evolves.

Although meta-analysis was somewhat slow to permeate into epidemiology, it has gathered a great deal of momentum since the mid 1980s. With the enthusiasm for meta-analysis has also come an increased debate around the proper use of meta-analysis and how to do them. It is likely that in future years, the science of meta-analysis will continue to evolve.

References

Berlin JA, Longnecker MP and Greenland S. Meta-analysis of epidemiologic dose-response data. 1993;4: 218–228.

Fleiss JL and Gross AJ. Meta-analysis in epidemiology, with special reference to studies on the association between exposure to environmental tobacco smoke and lung cancer: a critique. J Clin Epidemiol 1991;44:127–139.

Fleiss JL. The statistical basis of meta-analysis. Stat Methods Med Res 1993;2:121–145.

Friedenreich C. Methods for pooled analyses of epidemiologic studies. Epidemiology 1993;4:295–302.

Furberg CT and Morgan TM. Lessons from the overviews of cardiovascular trials. Stat Med 1987;6:295–303.

Glass GV. Primary, secondary, and meta-analysis of research. Educ Res 1976;5:3–8.

Greenland S. Quantitative methods in the review of epidemiologic literature. Epidemiol Rev 1987;91:30.

Greenland S and Longnecker MP. Methods for trend estimation from summarized dose-response data, with applications to meta-analysis. Am J Epidemiol 1992;135:1301–1309.

Greenland S. Invited commentary: A critical look at some popular meta-analytic methods. Am J Epidemiol 1994;140:290–296.

Griffith J, Aldrich T and Drane W. Risk assessment. In: Aldrich T, Griffith J (eds) Environmental Epidemiology and Risk Assessment. New York, NY: Van Nostrand Reinhold, 1993;212–239.

Hedges LV and Olkin I. Statistical Methods for Meta-Analysis. Orlando, FL: Academic Press, 1985.

Jenicek M. Meta-analysis in medicine: where we are and where we want to go. J Clin Epidemiol 1989;42:35–44.

L'Abbé KA, Detsky AS and O'Rourke K. Meta-analysis in clinical research. Ann Int Med 1987;107: 224–233.

Ladou J. The practice of occupational medicine. In: Ladou J (ed) Occupational Medicine. East Norwalk, CN: Appleton & Lange, 1990;1–4.

Laird NM and Mosteller F. Some statistical methods for combining experimental results. Int J Technol

Assessment Health Care 1990;6:5–30.

MacClure M. Demonstration of deductive meta-analysis: ethanol intake and risk of infarction. Epidemiol Rev 1993;15:328–351.

National Institutes of Health. Report of the National Institute of Health Ad Hoc Working Group to Develop Radioepidemiological Tables. U.S. Department of Health and Human Services, Washington DC, NIH 85–2748, 1985.

National Research Council, Commission on Life Sciences, Committee on the Institutional Means for Assessment of Risks to Public Health. Risk Assessment in the Federal Government: Managing the Process. Washington DC: National Academy Press, 1983.

National Research Council, Committee on the Biological Effects of Ionizing Radiation (BEIR). Health Risks of Radon and Other Internally Deposited Alpha-Emitters. Washington DC: National Academy Press, 1988;602.

Nicholson WJ. Quantitative risk assessment for carcinogens. In: Rom WN (ed) Environmental and Occupational Medicine. Second Edition. Boston, MA: Little, Brown and Company, 1992;1493.

O'Rourke K and Detsky AS. Meta-analysis in medical research: Strong encouragement for higher quality individual research efforts. J Clin Epidemiol 1989;42:1021–1029.

Petitti DB. Meta-Analysis, Decision Analysis and Cost-Effectiveness Analysis. New York, NY: Oxford University Press, Inc, 1994;246.

Rosenthal R. Meta-analysis: a review. Psychosomatic Med 1991;53:247–271.

Sacks HS, Berrier J, Reitman D, Ancona-Berk VA and Chalmers TC. Meta-analyses of randomized controlled trials. N Engl J Med 1987;316:450–455.

Spitzer WO. Meta-meta-analysis: unanswered questions about aggregating data. J Clin Epidemiol 1991;44:103–107.

Thacker SB. Meta-analysis: A quantitative approach to research integration. JAMA 1988;259:1685–1689.

Thompson SG and Pocock SJ. Can meta-analyses be trusted? Lancet 1991;338:1127–1130.

©1995 Elsevier Science B.V. All rights reserved.
The Role of Epidemiology in Regulatory Risk Assessment
J.D. Graham, editor.

How to use both human and animal data in quantitative risk assessment

Robert L. Sielken Jr

Sielken Inc., Bryan, Texas, USA

Abstract. Weight-of-evidence-based distributional characterizations of risk provide extensive opportunities for incorporating both human and animal data. This methodology is designed to reflect the current state of knowledge and all of the available, relevant information (including both human and animal data). The methodology is also a means of implementing a tiered approach to quantitative risk assessment by providing an unbiased, more realistic, and more comprehensive tier to follow a screening tier.

Human epidemiological data can provide additional alternatives for several of the factors in the probability tree for a risk assessment and hence be explicitly incorporated into the weight-of-evidence analysis. These alternatives have become increasingly meaningful and practical with the increasing availability of more and better exposure data and computer tools for the quantitative dose-response modeling of human epidemiological data.

Human epidemiological data and other human data can also help determine the relative weights on different alternatives in the analyses of animal data. In addition, these human data can be used to lessen the impact of methodological flaws and weaknesses in animal-based predictions of human risks.

Key words: assessment, bias, epidemiology, exposure, methodology, quantitative, risk.

Introduction

There are currently several significant opportunities to make much greater use of human data and especially human epidemiological data in quantitative risk assessments. This paper focuses on the opportunities in the dose-response and risk characterization portions of quantitative cancer risk assessments. There are also opportunities for greater use of human data in the qualitative hazard assessment portion of cancer risk assessment and several portions of noncancer risk assessment including the determinations of no-observed-adverse-effect-levels (NOAELs), lowest-observed-adverse-effect-levels (LOAELs), and benchmark doses as well as uncertainty factors like those for intraspecies variability and interspecies extrapolation. Exposure assessment is also not discussed herein, although greater use of human data in this area could substantially improve quantitative risk assessment. For example, human-data-based probability distribution characterizations of exposure model components or exposure equation components could provide much more information about the distribution of exposure in a population and even the 95th percentile of exposure than

Address for correspondence: Robert L. Sielken Jr, Sielken Inc., 3833 Texas Avenue, Suite 230, Bryan, TX 77802, USA. Tel.: +1-409–846–5175. Fax: +1-409–846–2671.

computations based on reasonable maximum exposures (RMEs).

The presentation of new approaches and tools is emphasized. The paper does not contain a comprehensive review of the literature.

The time is ripe to make more use of human epidemiological data. There are more human epidemiological data available than ever before with even more in the pipeline. These epidemiological data are accompanied by more exposure data, both in the form of direct (e.g., monitoring) data and indirect (e.g., biomarker) data. The emerging weight-of-evidence analysis methodology provides numerous opportunities to use both human data and animal data together in the dose-response and risk characterizations (Evans et al., 1994a and 1994b). The increased use of human epidemiological data are also facilitated by the increase in computer tools for dose-response modeling with epidemiological data. There are also new ways to incorporate human data into the interspecies extrapolation of animal-based human risk predictions. The time is also ripe because the need is so great.

Combining human epidemiological data with animal data in a weight-of-evidence-based distributional characterization of risk

Weight-of-evidence-based distributional characterizations of risk

Weight-of-evidence analyses are emerging as an alternative to the screening type of analyses frequently performed by federal regulatory agencies in which the quantitative dose-response assessment is dominated by default assumptions and limited to a single number, an upper bound on the cancer potency based solely on a single dose scale, a single dose-response model, a single data set, and a single method of interspecies extrapolation. These screening analyses ignore alternative dose scales, alternative dose-response models, alternative data sets, alternative methods of interspecies extrapolation, and alternative descriptions of the cancer potency, such as maximum likelihood estimates and bootstrap distributions of maximum likelihood estimates reflecting experimental variability rather than only an upper bound determined by a single computational methodology. In contrast, weight-of-evidence analyses consider all of the relevant alternatives, utilize all of the available and relevant information concerning an adverse health effect, and reflect the current state of knowledge rather than a single set of assumptions.

Weight-of-evidence analyses utilize a "tree" to explicitly identify the alternatives for each component factor in the risk assessment. For example, the tree in Fig. 1 corresponds to a very simplified assessment in which there are only three factors (dose scale, dose-response model, and data set) and only two alternatives for each factor. The two alternatives for the dose scale factor are: 1) use physiologically based pharmacokinetic (PBPK) modeling to determine the dose delivered to the target tissue and 2) assume that the delivered dose is proportional to the applied dose and do not use PBPK modeling. The dose-response modeling factor has two alternatives: 1) use a multistage model such as is often done with bioassay data, 2) use a proportional

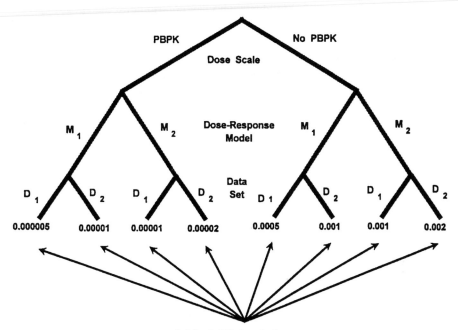

Fig. 1. Example tree.

hazards model which is a flexible model often used with epidemiological data. The two alternatives for the third factor are 1) a human epidemiological data set, and 2) an animal bioassay data set.

In a tree such as that displayed in Fig. 1, the alternatives are often referred to as "branches", and a "path" through the tree is a connected sequence of branches starting at the top of the tree and comprised of one branch for each factor. In this example tree there are eight paths; namely, (1,1,1), (1,1,2), (1,2,1), (1,2,2), (2,1,1), (2,1,2), (2,2,1), and (2,2,2) where (i,j,k) corresponds to the path with alternative i for the first factor, alternative j for the second factor, and alternative k for the third factor. Each path through the tree corresponds to an analysis.

The currently frequent practice of considering only one default alternative for each factor corresponds to considering only one path through the tree and ignoring the other paths. At the bottom of the tree at the end of each path is the risk characterization corresponding to that analysis, for example, the single number or distributional characterization of the added risk at a specified exposure level. Instead of basing the quantitative risk assessment on only a single path and its risk characterization, the weight-of-evidence approach explicitly identifies each of the alternatives for each factor and calculates the risk characterization for each combination of alternatives (i.e., for each path). Thus, the weight-of-evidence approach encourages a structural decomposition of the quantitative risk assessment, facilitates the involvement of individuals who can contribute to the specific parts of the assessment corresponding to their areas of expertise, and explicitly indicates the quantitative impact of alternatives.

In the tree, some of the paths and their corresponding analyses may be more plausible than other paths. Some paths may have stronger support from the relevant scientific communities. Hence, in the weight-of-evidence approach each of the alternatives for each factor on each path is assigned a weight such as in Fig. 2. The weight for an alternative is the relative emphasis given to that alternative (relative compared to the other alternatives) when all of the analyses are combined to generate the human risk characterization corresponding to the current state of knowledge. The weight for a specific alternative on a particular path may depend on the path's alternatives for the preceding factors. Thus, a weight acts like a conditional probability.

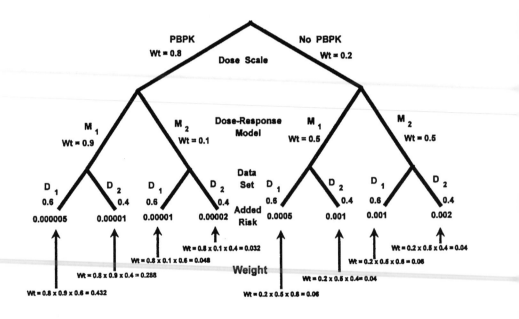

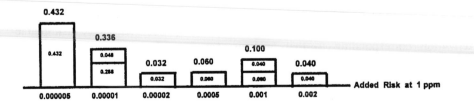

Fig. 2. Example tree. The most plausible added risk at 1 ppm is 0.000005 which has a relative likelihood of 43.2%.

Weights are numbers between 0.0 and 1.0, and at the end of each branch on each path the weights for the alternatives for the next factor sum to 1.0. For example, in Fig. 2, the weights for the two dose-scale alternatives are 0.8 and 0.2 which sum to 1.0 and indicate that, within the current state of knowledge, the first alternative (use PBPK modeling, "PBPK") is 4 times more plausible than the second alternative (do not use PBPK modeling, "No PBPK"). On the PBPK path, the weights for the two dose-response modeling alternatives are 0.9 and 0.1 which sum to 1.0 and indicate that the first alternative (proportional hazards modeling, "M_1") is currently 9 times more plausible than the second alternative multistage modeling, "M_2") when the dose scale is based on PBPK modeling. Finally, on the PBPK-M_1 path, the weights for the two data set alternatives are 0.6 and 0.4 which sum to 1.0 and indicate that the first alternative (an epidemiological data set, "D_1") is 1.5 times more plausible than the second alternative (a bioassay data set, "D_2") when the dose scale is based on PBPK modeling and the proportional hazards model is used for dose-response modeling.

The weight for a path and the risk characterization at the end of the path is the product of the weights (conditional probabilities) for the branches (alternatives) along the path, as illustrated in Fig. 2. The total weight on a particular risk characterization value is the sum of the weights over all paths that lead to that particular risk characterization value; hence, the weight on a particular risk comes from all analyses that predict that risk. The sum of the weights over all of the different risk characterizations is 1.0. The distribution of weight on different risks is a distributional characterization of risk indicating the relative plausibility of different values for the human risk under the current state of knowledge.

Example factors and alternatives in trees combining both human and animal data

One of the major advantages of the weight-of-evidence approach is that, by explicitly incorporating multiple alternatives for a factor and weighting each alternative according to its current relative plausibility, the approach can explicitly reflect the uncertainty in the current state of knowledge concerning the carcinogenic risk associated with a substance. For instance, a substance's carcinogenic mechanism may not be known for certain, so the tree incorporates the current possibilities (e.g., genotoxicity, cytotoxicity, and a combination of genotoxicity and cytotoxicity), and the weights for the alternatives reflect their relative support in the scientific community. The possibility of fractional weights, instead of all 0s and one 1, means that an alternative can be considered even though it has not been "proven" that the alternative is right and a default alternative is wrong. Such flexibility is important when such proofs are very rare.

The trees in Figs. 1 and 2 indicate only a few possible factors and a few alternatives for each factor. Fig. 3 expands the list of potential factors and alternatives in order to provide a better indication of the richness of the possibilities and the potential of the weight-of-evidence approach to encompass case-specific factors and alternatives. Of course, the list in Fig. 3 is not exhaustive, and in each specific case the final tree would usually focus on the most significant factors and alternatives.

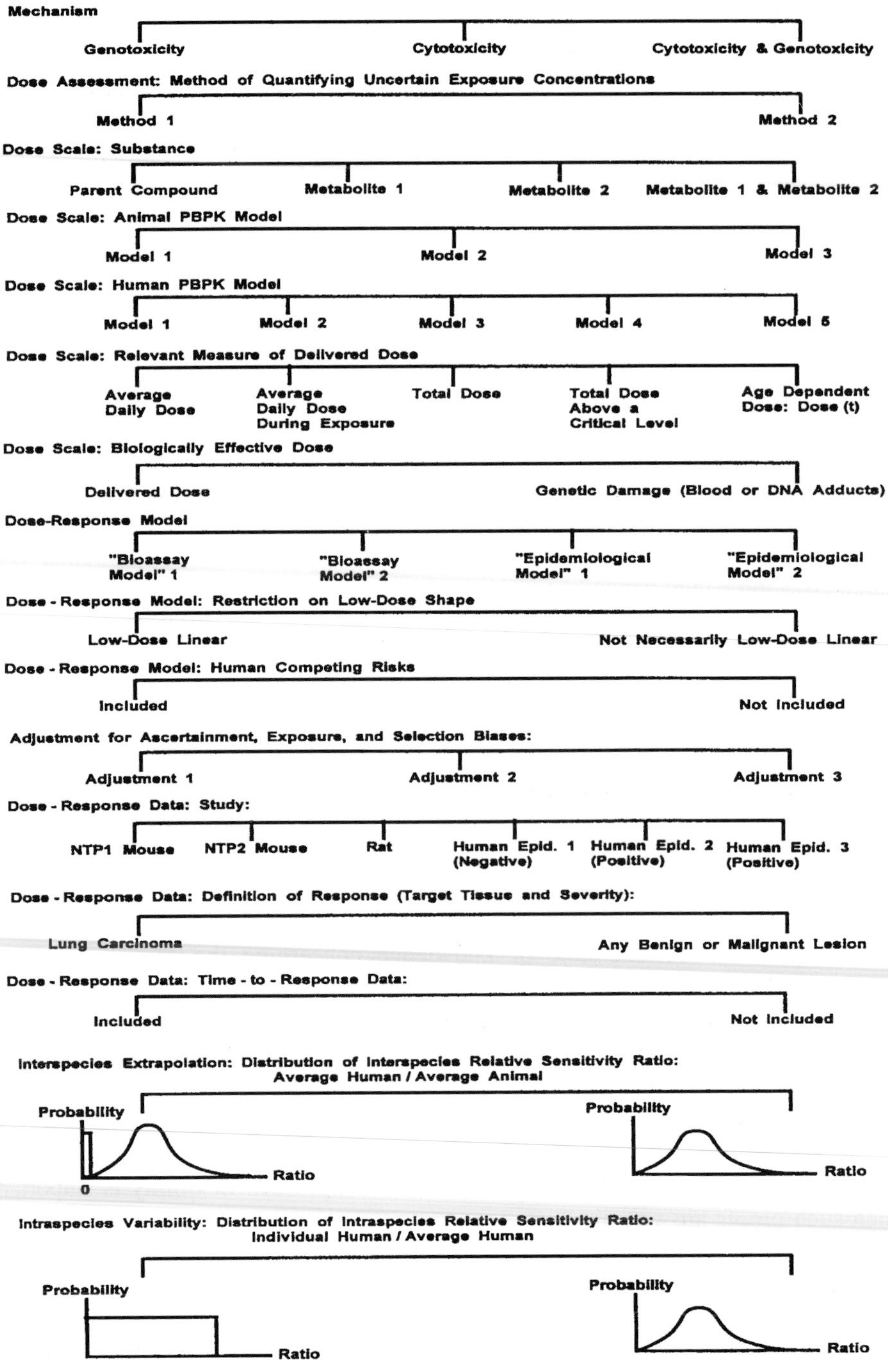

Mechanism

Genotoxicity   Cytotoxicity   Cytotoxicity & Genotoxicity

Dose Assessment: Method of Quantifying Uncertain Exposure Concentrations

Method 1   Method 2

Dose Scale: Substance

Parent Compound   Metabolite 1   Metabolite 2   Metabolite 1 & Metabolite 2

Dose Scale: Animal PBPK Model

Model 1   Model 2   Model 3

Dose Scale: Human PBPK Model

Model 1   Model 2   Model 3   Model 4   Model 5

Dose Scale: Relevant Measure of Delivered Dose

Average Daily Dose   Average Daily Dose During Exposure   Total Dose   Total Dose Above a Critical Level   Age Dependent Dose: Dose (t)

Dose Scale: Biologically Effective Dose

Delivered Dose   Genetic Damage (Blood or DNA Adducts)

Dose-Response Model

"Bioassay Model" 1   "Bioassay Model" 2   "Epidemiological Model" 1   "Epidemiological Model" 2

Dose - Response Model: Restriction on Low-Dose Shape

Low-Dose Linear   Not Necessarily Low-Dose Linear

Dose - Response Model: Human Competing Risks

Included   Not Included

Adjustment for Ascertainment, Exposure, and Selection Biases:

Adjustment 1   Adjustment 2   Adjustment 3

Dose - Response Data: Study:

NTP1 Mouse   NTP2 Mouse   Rat   Human Epid. 1 (Negative)   Human Epid. 2 (Positive)   Human Epid. 3 (Positive)

Dose - Response Data: Definition of Response (Target Tissue and Severity):

Lung Carcinoma   Any Benign or Malignant Lesion

Dose - Response Data: Time - to - Response Data:

Included   Not Included

Interspecies Extrapolation: Distribution of Interspecies Relative Sensitivity Ratio: Average Human / Average Animal

Probability — Ratio 0   Probability — Ratio

Intraspecies Variability: Distribution of Intraspecies Relative Sensitivity Ratio: Individual Human / Average Human

Probability — Ratio   Probability — Ratio

Fig. 3. Example factors and alternatives in a tree combining both human and animal data.

Trees combining both human and animal data

Human epidemiological data and the dose-response modeling of that data can be explicitly incorporated into the probability tree and its resultant distributional characterization of human risks. In this approach the epidemiological data sets, the types of dose-response models used for modeling epidemiological data, etc. are explicitly included among the alternatives for the factors in the probability tree.

The probability tree is not divided into an animal tree and a human tree. The animal and human alternatives for each factor are considered as a single set of alternatives. Some factors may not affect all analyses; so that, on some paths the alternatives for a specific factor may not alter the risk characterization and the weight on that analysis's risk characterization is unaffected by the weights on the different alternatives for that specific factor. For example, a factor may only apply to animal data or only apply to human data (e.g., interspecies extrapolation, confounding exposures, and length of follow-up are factors which sometimes only apply to one type of data).

New methods of dose-response modeling with human epidemiological data

Quantified human exposures allow explicit dose-response modeling of human epidemiological data in addition to the more classical epidemiological comparisons between exposed and unexposed populations and "positive" or "negative" findings. Also, the emergence of more and better human exposure data and the increased opportunities to include the results of the dose-response modeling of human epidemiological data into the quantitative risk assessment through weight-of-evidence analyses are encouraging the continued development of more methods of dose-response modeling that can be applied to human epidemiological data.

There are now a wide variety of fairly new methods of quantitative dose-response modeling that can be applied to human epidemiological data. For instance, the statistical and computer tools have been extended to enable the same dose-response models that have been used to do high-to-low-dose extrapolations with animal bioassay data to be fit to human epidemiological data and serve as a basis for human dose-response predictions. The GEN.T software provided by Sielken, Inc., is one such (GEN)eral (T)ool for fitting dose-response models and making dose-response inferences using either quantal models which ignore time-to-response information or time-to-response models. Among the quantal models are the probit, logit, Weibull, multihit, multistage, and linearized multistage models. Among the time-to-response models are multistage-Weibull, Weibull-Weibull, Hartley-Sielken, Armitage-Doll, two-stage growth (Suresh Moolgavkar et al.), and Gompertz-Makeham models. K.S. Crump & Company also provides some dose-response modeling software.

Animal bioassay data are often treated as grouped data with only a few dose levels (e.g., 50 animals at the maximum tolerated dose (MTD), 50 animals at one-half the MTD, 50 animals at one-quarter of the MTD, and 50 control animals). Human epidemiological data are sometimes treated as grouped data with only a few dose levels. Any dose-response model and modeling tools capable of analyzing animal bioassay data can be used to analyze this type of grouped human epidemiological data. However, human epidemiological data often have many individuals with different dose levels because of differences in exposure start and stop times, exposure levels during times of exposure, occupational histories, etc. Fortunately, such data do not necessarily have to be treated as grouped data with only a few dose levels. Special tools are available to treat data with a large number of dose levels including cases where essentially each exposed individual has a unique dose level. For example, EPID.T is an extension of GEN.T designed to fit data with a large number of dose levels or even unique individual dose levels and to make dose-response predictions.

The types of dose-response models usually applied to animal bioassay data can now also be considered for human epidemiological data, and vice versa, some of the types of dose-response models applied to human epidemiological data can also be applied to animal bioassay data. An advantage of using the same family of dose-response models for both human and animal data are that the estimated dose dependence of each parameter or component in the animal-based model can be directly compared to the estimated dose dependence of the same parameter or component in the human-based model. This sometimes highlights interspecies differences in the dose-response relationships for a substance and may suggest mechanistic differences.

There are new software tools that expand the dose-response modeling of human epidemiological data by allowing age-dependent dose levels instead of lifetime average daily doses or other averages. Some dose-response modeling software, such as GEN.T and EPID.T, can explicitly incorporate age-dependent doses; that is, doses where the dose level is a function of time rather than just a single number representation of a history of dose levels like total dose or lifetime average daily dose. This currently, mostly unused capability should be important in modeling human occupational exposures in which the dose level is hardly ever constant over time and even in modeling animal experimental data where exposures are not always at a constant level. This capability should also be important in biologically based dose-response models which model cancer as a process that evolves over the lifetime of the individual rather than an instantaneous event.

There are new software tools and analytical methods that facilitate dose-response modeling with human epidemiological data by expanding the set of possible dose-response models. In addition to the tools that allow for the use of the dose-response models that are usually applied to animal bioassay data, some general statistical techniques such as regression analysis can be used to do dose-response modeling with human epidemiological data. More advanced statistical techniques such as nonlinear regression analysis, Poisson regression, and proportional hazards models can also be used.

Proportional hazards models offer a special advantage in that they can directly incorporate a given (known or assumed) background hazard rate and its age dependence. In a proportional hazards model,

$$\text{Hazard rate} = [\text{Background population hazard rate}] \times [\exp\{\beta_1 Z_1 + \beta_2 Z_2 + \dots + \beta_k Z_k\}]$$

where Z_1, Z_2, ... are covariates and β_1, β_2,... are coefficients to be estimated. The covariates can be functions of dose such as total dose in a lifetime, lifetime average daily dose, average dose during exposure period, etc. or refer to occupational history such as age at start of employment or duration of employment or refer to some other potentially important characteristics such as gender, medical history, smoking habits, etc. Furthermore, some computer implementations of the proportional hazard model allow for age-dependent covariates so that the possibilities for covariates can be extended to include age-specific doses, age-dependent total doses, age-dependent employment duration, etc.

Modeling tools that can include covariates are especially important when modeling human data because the variability in human situations and characteristics may be considerably greater than that of experimental animals.

Using human data on a specific substance to help weight alternatives in animal-based predictions of the substance's human risk

Human data can help determine the weights on the different alternatives for several of the factors in a probability tree analysis of different animal-based predictions of human risk and, thereby, significantly impact the resulting distributional characterization of the plausibility of different human risks. For example, human epidemiological data can help determine the weight on alternative animal data sets with different target organs, alternative animal data sets with different routes of exposure, alternative characterizations of the human background response probability, and alternative characterizations of the relative sensitivity of humans compared to different animal species.

Human pharmacokinetic data can help determine weights on the alternative dose scales used for animal dose-response modeling by indicating if and how well different measures of human delivered doses (target tissue doses) can be determined, and, hence, how useful interspecies extrapolations of risk on delivered dose scales will be for predicting human risks. The usefulness of predictions on the delivered dose scale depends on the ability to transform the risks back to risks in terms of exposure media concentrations.

Human in vivo and in vitro studies at low doses of events related to the carcinogenic process can help determine weights on the alternative restrictions on the low-dose shape in dose-response models used for high-to-low-dose extrapolation.

Human pharmacodynamic studies can help determine the weights on the alternative characterizations of the relative sensitivity of humans compared to animals and, hence, help determine the weights on the alternative methods of interspecies extrapolation.

Human studies on interindividual variability in background doses and susceptibility and their distributions in different target populations can help determine the weights on the alternative characterizations of interindividual variability and the relative sensitivity of individual humans compared to the average human and, hence, help determine the weights on the alternative methods of interspecies extrapolation.

There is a need for methodology to make the impact of human epidemiology data and other forms of human data on the weights for the alternatives in animal-based predictions of human risk explicit and quantifiable. The elicitation and use of expert judgements based on both human and animal data are an emerging possibility. More experience and examples are needed.

Using human epidemiological data on several substances to help weight alternatives in animal-based predictions of a different substance's human risk

The preceding section discusses a method of combining the animal data on a specified substance with the human data on that same specified substance. This section discusses a method of combining the animal data on a specified substance with the human epidemiological data on substances other than the specified substance.

Human epidemiological data on substances other than the specific substance under study can be used to improve the specific substance's weight-of-evidence-based distributional characterization of human risk by identifying the weights that performed best in predicting the human risks for these other substances from animal data. The basic idea is that new predictions are more likely to be better if they use weights that worked well in the past. EXTRACT is a computer tool written by Sielken Inc, with support from the American Industrial Health Council (AIHC) and utilizing the historical database assembled by K.S. Crump & Company for their "Investigation of Cancer Risk Assessment Methods", facilitating the determination of the weights on alternatives that perform best on a historical database or perform best on a user-specified subset of substances in this database. The database contains human epidemiological data for the 23 substances identified in Fig. 4 and, for each substance, a large set of animal-based predictions of human risk. The set of animal-based predictions corresponds to all of the relevant combinations of the different alternatives for the 11 different factors indicated in Fig. 5. By **EX**amining **T**he **R**isk Assessment Components **T**ogether, EXTRACT can enable a weight-of-evidence analysis to weight most heavily the alternatives that perform the best in a statistical analysis of "observed" human risk based on human epidemiological data versus "predicted" human risk based on animal data. EXTRACT is an example of computer software that utilizes a historical database to compare and quantify the performance of different methods of predicting human risks from animal data, and then utilizes the relative performances of different methods to generate weights for those methods on the basis of their demonstrated ability to predict human risks from animal data. Such software could be expanded to include additional substances as well as additional factors and alternatives. This method of utilizing human epidemiological data to obtain weights on alternative procedures for generating animal-based predictions of human risks is another method of combining both human and animal data in a quantitative risk assessment.

Industrial chemical	Food additive or contaminant
Arsenic	Saccharin
Asbestos	
Benzene	Aflatoxin
Benzidene	
Chromium	
Vinyl chloride	Drug
Epichlorohydrin	Chlorambucil
Ethylene oxide	Diethylstilbestrol
Methylene chloride	Estrogens
Polychlorinated biphenyls	Melphalan
Trichloroethylene	Phenacetin
Nickel	Isoniazid
Cadmium	Reserpine
	Other
	Cigarette smoke

Fig. 4. In EXTRACT, performance is evaluated in terms of the ability of the combination of factor alternatives to predict the human dose with a 25% response rate from animal data in a user-specified subset of the 23 trial cases corresponding to the following 23 substances.

Combining data on the human condition with animal data to improve animal-based predictions of human risks

There are at least five types of human data that can be used to improve the interspecies extrapolation of animal-based dose-response modeling results. These five types of human data are:
1) human competing risks,
2) human background parameter values,
3) human background dose levels,
4) human pharmacokinetics and pharmacodynamics, and
5) the distribution of human susceptibility values and background doses.

Some of these human data, such as the human pharmacokinetic and pharmacodynamic data, may not be "epidemiological data" in the classical sense; however, there is such an underappreciated need and opportunity to utilize these data to improve the animal-based predictions of human risks that they have been included in this discussion of how to use both human and animal data in risk assessment.

These human data make possible improvements or corrections in the interspecies extrapolation of risks, the use of more relevant dose scales for animal dose-response modeling, and the expansion of risk predictions to include more interindividual variability.

Factor 1.	Length of experiment
	Alternative a. Use data from any experiment but correct for short observation periods.
	Alternative b. Use data from experiments which last no less than 90% of the standard length of the experiment.
Factor 2.	Length of dosing
	Alternative a. Use data from any experiment, regardless of exposure duration.
	Alternative b. Use data from experiments that expose animals to the test chemical no less than 80% of the standard experiment length.
Factor 3.	Route of exposure
	Alternative a. Use data from experiment for which route of exposure is most similar to that encountered by humans.
	Alternative b. Use data from any experiment, regardless of route of exposure.
	Alternative c. Use data from experiments that exposed animals by gavage, inhalation, any oral route, or the route most similar to that encountered by humans.
Factor 4.	Dose units assumed to give human-animal equivalence
	Alternative a. mg/kg body wt/day.
	Alternative b. ppm in diet.
	Alternative c. ppm in air.
	Alternative d. mg/kg body wt/lifetime.
	Alternative e. mg/m^2 surface area/day.
Factor 5.	Calculation of average dose
	Alternative a. Doses expressed as average dose up to termination of experiment.
	Alternative b. Doses expressed as average dose over the first 80% of the experiment.
Factor 6.	Animals to use in analysis
	Alternative a. Use all animals for the particular tumor type.
	Alternative b. Use animals surviving just prior to discovery of the first tumor of the type chosen.
Factor 7.	Malignancy status to consider
	Alternative a. Consider malignant tumors only.
	Alternative b. Consider both benign and malignant tumors.
Factor 8.	Particular tumor type to use
	Alternative a. Use combination of tumor types with significant dose-response.
	Alternative b. Use total tumor-bearing animals.
	Alternative c. Use response that occurs in humans.
	Alternative d. Use any individual response.

Fig. 5. Factors and alternatives that can be evaluated in EXTRACT.

Factor 9.	Combining data from males and females
	Alternative a. Use data from each sex within a study separately.
	Alternative b. Average results for different sexes within a study.
Factor 10.	Combining data from different studies
	Alternative a. Consider every study within species separately.
	Alternative b. Average the results of different studies.
Factor 11.	Combining data from different studies
	Alternative a. Combine results from all available species.
	Alternative b. Combine results from mice and rats.
	Alternative c. Use data from a single preselected species.
	Alternative d. Consider all species separately.

Fig. 5. (Continued)

Using human epidemiological data to lessen the impact of methodological flaws and weaknesses in animal-based predictions of human risks

Incorporating human competing risks

Human epidemiological data on competing risks can be incorporated into the interspecies extrapolation of animal-based dose-response models, instead of falsely assuming that human competing risks are absent or the same as the competing risks for experimental animals. Competing risks are all hazards other than the specified hazard of concern. For example, if lung cancer is the specified hazard, then heart disease and prostrate cancer are two of the many competing risks. The current time-to-response model predictions of the probability of a specified response during a specified time period, like 70 years, omit all competing risks and, hence, overpredict the risk because competing risks may prevent an individual from being at risk for the entire specified period. Quantal response models (e.g., probit, multistage, and multihit models) implicitly assume that the human competing risks are the same as the competing risks in the experimental situation, usually experimental animals. These weaknesses can be overcome by using cause-specific modeling which explicitly includes the hazard rate for competing risks as well as the hazard rate for the specified response (Kalbfleisch et al., 1983). Computer software for dose-response models incorporating competing risks or cause-specific modeling are not readily available but could be developed by extending existing software.

Incorporating human background parameter values

Human epidemiological data can be used to estimate the human background response probability and other human background parameters that can facilitate the extrapolation of animal-based dose-response models to humans.

A frequently occurring flaw in current animal-based risk assessments is that, while "added" or "extra" risks do reflect the incremental risk above the background risk, the usual estimates and bounds for the slope of these risks vs. dose in multistage and linearized multistage models, respectively, do not correctly reflect the interspecies differences in the background transition rates between stages in an underlying multistage carcinogenic process. The human background response probability can be used to at least heuristically correct for this flaw and improve the multistage model estimates of the human cancer potency and linearized multistage model upper bounds on the human cancer potency (Sielken and Stevenson, 1994).

The human background mutation rates, cell birth and death rates, etc. can be used in the interspecies extrapolation of two stage growth models such as those developed by Suresh Moolgavkar et al.

Incorporating human background dose values

Human data on the background dose allows the differences between the background level in humans and animals to be incorporated into interspecies extrapolations of animal-based dose-response models. This avoids the mathematical flaw in interspecies extrapolations corresponding to the unfortunately common use of "human equivalent doses" in dose-response modeling (Sielken, 1989).

Frequently, humans are assumed to be more sensitive than animals by some interspecies scaling factor, say FACTOR. Then, the human potency is determined by dividing the animal doses by FACTOR to form so-called "human equivalent doses" (HEDs). The human dose-response model is then supposedly obtained by fitting the animal response frequencies to the human equivalent dose levels. If the human background dose level is not equal to the animal background level divided by FACTOR and the dose-response relationship is not linear over its entire range, then the human cancer potency based on the use of HEDs is mathematically incorrect. Here, background dose level includes not only the background dose of the substance being evaluated but also the background level of the type of mechanistic activity associated with that substance regardless of whether or not the background level of activity is caused by the specific substance, other substances, or other processes.

The correct procedure is to do the dose-response modeling by fitting the animal response frequencies to the animal dose levels on a biologically effective dose scale which includes the effects of both the background dose and the administered or applied dose. Then estimate the human response probability at a biologically effective dose (BED) equal to BED* to be the animal response probability at a biologically effective dose BED* × FACTOR. The terminology, biologically effective dose, is used to indicate a dose scale that may incorporate, in addition to the delivery process, the net effects of the biological processes like cell proliferation and DNA adduct formation and repair that take place after the delivered dose has arrived at the target tissue. The biologically effective dose indicates a biologically operative dose but not necessarily a dose level guaranteed to cause cancer.

Of course, another use of both human epidemiological data and animal data in quantitative risk assessment is to use such paired data on substances that are "similar" to the substance under study to estimate FACTOR.

Using human data to improve interspecies extrapolation of animal-based dose-response modeling results

Incorporating more biologically relevant dose scales

Human pharmacokinetic and pharmacodynamic data allow interspecies extrapolation of dose-response models with more biologically relevant dose scales. Dose-response modeling with more biologically relevant dose scales allows the high-to-low-dose extrapolations to reflect more of available and relevant biological and mechanistic information in the experimental species. The human pharmacokinetic and pharmacodynamic data allow the interspecies extrapolation of dose-response models with more biologically relevant dose scales to reflect the interspecies differences in the corresponding pharmacokinetic and pharmacodynamic processes (Sielken, 1987; Lu and Sielken, 1991; Holland and Sielken, 1993; and many others).

Part of the evolution in dose-response modeling has been the increased use of more biologically relevant dose scales. For example, if the dose scale used for dose-response modeling is INTAKE rather than simply media CONCENTRATION, then not only does the animal dose-response modeling incorporate the available information relating animal intake and media concentration but also, when the risk is extrapolated from animals to humans on the intake scale and the risk on the human intake scale subsequently transformed into a risk on the media concentration scale, the available information relating human intake and media concentrations is incorporated. Furthermore, if the dose scale used for dose-response modeling is a DELIVERED DOSE rather than just INTAKE, then the available information in both humans and animals relating the amount of intake to the amount of the substance or its active metabolite delivered to the target tissue is also incorporated. Even better, if the dose scale used for dose-response modeling is a BIOLOGICALLY EFFECTIVE DOSE rather than just DELIVERED DOSE, then the available information in both humans and animals relating the amount of substance delivered to the target tissue to the net amount of relevant biological activity generated within the target tissue (e.g., DNA adducts not repaired or cell regeneration) is also incorporated. Hence, the dose scale represents a conduit for incorporating a tremendous amount of biological information on both humans and animals.

As suggested in Fig. 6, the use of more biologically relevant dose scales allows for the incorporation of more human data on susceptibility and background dose as well as pharmacokinetics, pharmacodynamics, differences between exposure routes, and dose-rate effects when the dose is not constant over time.

Incorporating interindividual variability

Data on the distribution of human background dose and the distribution of susceptibility in humans can be used to explicitly incorporate at least some of the human interindividual variability into risk predictions (Holland and Sielken, 1993). The distribution of human background dose can reflect some of the interindividual variability in human exposures and the things such as lifestyle that may affect exposures. The distribution of susceptibility values can be used to explicitly

120

incorporate the variability in human physiological processes.

The interindividual variability reflected in the distributions of susceptibility and background dose can be incorporated into the characterization of the risk associated with a specified concentration of a substance in an exposure medium by calculating the risk not for a single value of the biologically effective dose corresponding to the specified media concentration and some average or default values for susceptibility and background dose but rather for the distribution of biologically effective dose values corresponding to the specified media concentration and the distribution of susceptibility and background dose values. The resulting distribution of risk values incorporates the interindividual variability in susceptibility and background dose.

Both GEN.T and EPID.T can incorporate distributions of susceptibility and background dose.

In addition to the human data on the distribution of susceptibility and background dose, the human data on the distributions of other relevant biological parameters in the target populations and subpopulations could also be explicitly incorporated into the estimation of the distribution of risks among individuals. Software could be expanded to incorporate distributions of human background mutation rates, cell birth and death rates, etc. into two stage growth models such as those developed by Suresh Moolgavkar et al. Similarly, current software could be expanded to incorporate

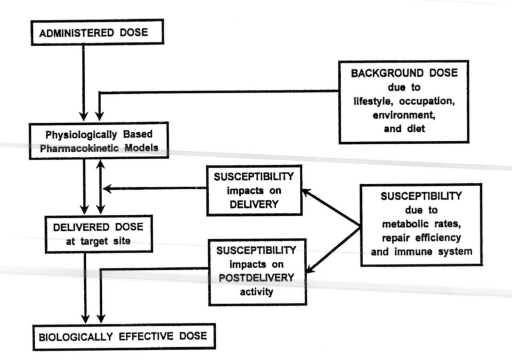

Fig. 6. Biologically effective dose as a function of administered dose, background dose, delivered dose and susceptibility.

distributions of the biological parameters in physiologically based pharmacokinetic (PBPK) models.

Consistency checks

In the past, the use of human epidemiological data has largely been restricted to so-called "consistency checks" on animal-based predictions of human risk. Unfortunately, this limits the use of human epidemiological data to either accepting or rejecting predicted risks. This limited use contrasts sharply with the role for human epidemiological data advanced in the preceding portions of this paper; namely, the role of actually predicting what the risks are or determining the likelihood of different values of the risk or performing these functions in combination with animal data. However, if human epidemiological data are going to be used to perform consistency checks, then there are sometimes better ways to do such checks.

Traditional consistency checks based on human epidemiological data have not been very powerful. If the animal-based predictions were to say that the cancer response probability would increase from a background level of P_0 to a value of $P_0 + q_1^* \times d$ at a dose d, then an enormous number (N) of people who actually had a cancer response probability of P_0 at dose d would have to be observed before there would even be a 50% chance that the 95% upper confidence limit on their cancer response probability was not as big as $P_0 + q_1^* \times d$. For example, if $P_0 = 0.01$ and $q_1^* \times d = 0.00001 = 1/100,000$, then N = 270,000,000. Consistency checks which attempt to reject a hypothesized nonzero cancer potency or added risk at moderate to low doses either by comparing a group of individuals at a constant dose level to a control group or by comparing the observed cancer frequency in a group of individuals at a constant dose to a hypothesized frequency have very little chance of success even when the true cancer potency is zero.

The shape of the dose-response model when it is fit to human epidemiological data can be the basis for more powerful consistency checks on animal-based predictions of human risk. In fact, the only type of consistency checks that may have any real chance of rejecting a hypothesized cancer potency or added risk that is too large are consistency checks based on dose-response modeling that attempt to reject false hypotheses on the basis of their inconsistency with the observed shape of the dose-response model.

In a recent analysis, a hypothesized human cancer potency (q_1^*) was rejected by determining that the likelihood was too small that the observed human epidemiological data could have arisen from a multistage dose-response model with added risks corresponding to a cancer potency as large as q_1^*. In this analysis, the relative likelihood of the observed human epidemiological data was determined at each point in the parameter space of the multistage model. The added risk (at 1 µg/kg/day) was also calculated at each possible point in the parameter space of the multistage model. The total likelihood on added risks as large as those implied by the hypothesized cancer potency (q_1^*) was less than 5% (in fact, less than 0.1%) of the total relative likelihood at all points in the parameter space of the multistage model. An interesting sidelight to this example consistency check was that the hypothesized value of q_1^* was only rejected when the underlying multistage model family was sufficiently flexible (had a sufficiently high degree polynomial in dose with parameters not restricted to all be nonnegative) to do a good job of reflecting the observed shape of the dose-response relationship in the human epidemiological data.

Discussion

There are at least two major ways that human epidemiological data can be combined with animal data in a weight-of-evidence-based distributional characterization of risk. One way is for the human epidemiological data and the dose-response modeling of that data to be explicitly incorporated into the probability tree and its resultant distributional characterization of human risks. A second way is to use the human epidemiological data to help determine the weights on the different alternatives for each factor in a probability tree analysis of different animal-based predictions of human risk and thereby significantly impact the resulting distributional characterization of the likelihood of different human risks.

Weight-of-evidence-based distributional characterization of risk provide opportunities to help build consensus and to include all of the available relevant information including both human and animal data and both positive and negative studies.

There are some significant challenges. One challenge is to continue to improve the methods of determining consensus weights, especially the elicitation and quantification of the weights corresponding to the current state of knowledge in the relevant scientific communities. Another challenge is to effectively communicate distributional characterizations to the public and other risk managers as well as to facilitate the use of distributional characterizations in their risk management decision making.

References

Evans JS, Gray GM, Sielken RL Jr, Smith AE, Valdez-Flores C and Graham JD. Use of probabilistic expert judgment in uncertainty analysis of carcinogenic potency. Regulatory Toxicology and Pharmacology 1994;20(1).

Evans JS, Graham JD, Gray GM and Sielken RL Jr. A distributional approach to characterizing low-dose cancer risk. Risk Analysis 1994b;14(1):25–34.

Holland CD and Sielken RL Jr. Cancer Modeling and Risk Assessment, New Jersey: Prentice Hall, Englewood Cliffs, 1993.

Kalbfleisch JD, Krewski D and Van Ryzin J. Dose response models for time to response toxicity data. Can J Stat 1983;11(1):25–49.

Lu FC and Sielken RL Jr. Assessment of safety/risk of chemicals: inception and evolution of the ADI and dose-response modeling procedures. Toxicol Lett 1991;59:5–40.

Sielken RL Jr. Cancer dose-response extrapolations. Environ Sci Technol 1987;21(11):1033–1039.

Sielken RL Jr and Smith LA. Cancer dose-response models. In: Hayes AW, Schnell RC and Miya TS (eds) Developments in the Science and Practice of Toxicology, 1983;173–180.

Sielken RL Jr and Stevenson DE. Comparison of human cancer potency projections for dieldrin based on human data with those based on animal data. In: D'Amato R, Slaga TJ, Farland WH and Henry C (eds) Relevance of Animal Studies to Evaluate Human Cancer Risk. New York: John Wiley & Sons, Inc., 1992;295–319.

Sielken RL Jr and Stevenson DE. Another flaw in the linearized multistage model upper bounds on human cancer potency. Reg Toxicol Pharmacol 1994;19(1):106–114.

Sielken RL Jr. GEN.T: a general tool for incorporating interspecies extrapolation information into quantitative cancer risk assessment. Proceedings of the 1989 ACT/SRA Workshop on Inferring Carcinogenic Effects in One Species from Data on a Different Species.

©1995 Elsevier Science B.V. All rights reserved.
The Role of Epidemiology in Regulatory Risk Assessment
J.D. Graham, editor.

Using both animal and human data in risk assessment: notes on current practice

Lorenz Rhomberg

Harvard Center for Risk Analysis, Boston, Massachusetts, USA

Key words: assessment, carcinogenicity, epidemiology, lifetime exposure, risk, toxicity.

I would like to review some current practices for using both epidemiological findings and the results of animal bioassays in regulatory risk assessment. I will stress the practices at the U.S. Environmental Protection Agency; assessment practices elsewhere are essentially similar, although they are sometimes less explicitly structured. Assessments at EPA are governed by formal guidelines (EPA, 1987a), providing a useful framework for setting out the various steps, identifying issues and questions, and making explicit the presumptions that are made in the face of inconclusive or conflicting results. (These guidelines are under revision; departures from current procedure that have been proposed (EPA, 1989; EPA, 1994) will be noted below). My comments will also focus on carcinogen risk assessment, but the principles apply with some modification to the assessment of noncancer toxicity as well.

Following the recommendations of the National Academy of Sciences' "Red Book" (NAS, 1983), a distinction is made between the qualitative question of whether an agent might be a human carcinogen (under some circumstances with some unspecified potency, which may be high or low) and the subsequent quantitative question of what magnitude of risk might be associated with different levels of exposure. Assessment of the evidence on the first — qualitative — question is termed hazard identification. Broadly speaking, this evidence can be classed into three categories:
 — epidemiological evidence,
 — the results of lifetime-exposure animal bioassays, and
 — a variety of ancillary evidence.
This last category includes various short-term tests (for genotoxicity, promotional activity, etc.), knowledge of the toxic properties of structurally analogous compounds, pharmacokinetics, and so on. In current EPA practice, these three categories are initially considered separately.

Address for correspondence: Lorenz Rhomberg, Harvard Center for Risk Analysis, 718 Huntington Avenue, Boston, MA 02115, USA. Tel.: +1-617-432-0095. Fax: +1-617-432-0190.

At least broadly, the nature of the transformation of normal cells to tumor cells and the elements of the carcinogenic process are thought to be similar among mammalian organisms. Thus, the demonstration of an agent's carcinogenicity in experimental rodent bioassays provides *prima facie* evidence that the agent might be a carcinogen in humans as well. This presumption can be questioned, but the first step is to examine the animal evidence to determine whether carcinogenicity has indeed been demonstrated. The details are beyond the scope of this paper, but an evaluation of the body of animal evidence is conducted that stresses good experimental practice, adequate study power, and the repeatability of results. The body of animal evidence collectively is then classified as either "sufficient," "limited," or "inadequate" for concluding that the agent is shown to be carcinogenic *in animal tests*.

A parallel analysis is conducted of the body of epidemiological evidence. The individual studies (if there are any, which is not always the case) are critically evaluated by agency epidemiologists for an assessment of study quality. This includes an evaluation of the soundness of study design, adequacy of the reporting and analysis of data, and an assessment of the potential roles of bias, confounding, and chance in determining the study's results. Many of the available studies for chemicals of interest to the EPA are occupational cohort studies, and the issues that typically arise in the interpretation of such studies must be dealt with. These include: the adequacy of exposure measures, their estimates or surrogates (including misclassification and the effects of aggregation); the possibility of coexposures to other potentially carcinogenic chemicals; the potential role of smoking as a confounder or effect modifier; and the comparability of control groups or reference populations to those exposed in all matters save exposure. For studies on potential carcinogens, one is particularly concerned that the duration of exposure is enough and follow-up is sufficiently long and complete so as to provide an adequate opportunity to observe any effects appearing late in life after chronic exposure. The aggregation of tumors of different histological types or anatomical sites, and the adequacy of identification of primary tumor types may also be an issue.

Once the available studies have been scrutinized individually, they are then evaluated collectively for the degree to which the body of evidence taken as a whole supports the interpretation of the substance as a causal agent of human cancer. This is no different from the process that any other epidemiologists would go through — the intent is to characterize the evidence for causality in a way that reflects good, informed epidemiological judgment according to the established criteria of the field. The Bradford Hill criteria serve as a guide; that is, in addition to the criteria by which individual studies are judged, the Agency also examines questions of coherence, consistency, and specificity that emerge when one simultaneously considers the outcomes of multiple studies. There is also the opportunity to address biological plausibility by bringing into consideration the results of the animal studies and various other information on pharmacokinetics and mechanism of toxic action.

By and large, this collective evaluation of the body of epidemiological evidence is done qualitatively, by argument and discussion of the evidence. In recent years, the field of epidemiology has explored the use of more quantitative approaches (meta-analysis, discussed elsewhere in this volume), and such analysis has figured in the recent EPA assessments of environmental tobacco smoke and oxides of Nitrogen (EPA, 1992, 1993).

In sum, then, the evaluation of epidemiological data are done according to the standards of the field. All of the discussions elsewhere in this volume about the use and interpretation of epidemiological studies apply. The principal additional consideration is that a regulatory agency must come to a fairly explicit "bottom line" conclusion about the evidence for causality. The body of epidemiological evidence is classified as "sufficient," "limited," or "inadequate." (As with the animal data, there are also categories for "no data" and "no evidence," i.e., evidence of noncarcinogenicity through lack of response in several well conducted, sufficiently powerful studies. This last category has been problematic, as will be discussed further below.)

The names of the weight-of-evidence categories are the same as those used for the animal data, but the question being asked is different — it is the question of causality in humans rather than of demonstration of the end point in animals. "Sufficient" evidence constitutes establishment of the agent's carcinogenicity in humans according to the criteria prevailing in the field. The "limited" evidence category comprises cases in which a causal interpretation is credible, but chance, bias, or confounding cannot be ruled out with confidence. Evidence is "inadequate" either when there are insufficient data or when chance, bias, or confounding are deemed to be more credible as explanations of the observed results than is the putative carcinogenicity of the agent.

Once these separate characterizations of the human and animal evidence have been produced, they are then combined into an overall "weight of evidence". (It is at this point that the "ancillary" evidence comes to bear, illuminating the appropriate synthesis of animal and human data by addressing questions of the commonality of underlying mechanisms.) If the evidence for carcinogenicity in humans is "stronger" than in animals, then the human evidence prevails. (It does after all directly address the primary question.) Agents with "sufficient" human evidence are categorized as "known" human carcinogens (Group A) regardless of the status of animal evidence. Similarly, agents with "limited" human evidence are always put in Group B1 (probable human carcinogen). From this point of view, the role of epidemiology in risk assessment could scarcely be stronger; it overrules all other considerations.

The interesting question — and the focus of the balance of this essay — arises for agents with rather strongly supported findings of carcinogenicity in animal tests and essentially "negative" results in the existing epidemiological studies. How should such results be combined?

Human studies are usually considered less powerful as detectors of carcinogenicity than are animal studies. There are several reasons for this. Firstly, the exposures available for study among human populations are generally lower than those used in rodent bioassays, often much lower. The possibility exists that tumors are being caused in humans, but (owing to the low exposure) at a lower rate than in animals, one that cannot statistically be distinguished from background but that nonetheless constitutes a public health concern. Unlike rodent bioassays, epidemiological studies also are generally of less-than-lifetime exposures and have less-than-lifetime follow-up, reducing their relative power to detect effects. Secondly, the issues of bias and confounding can rarely be totally dismissed in real-word situations, while animal studies avoid these issues through rigorous control of experimental conditions.

For all of these reasons, some epidemiologists resist calling a study "negative," preferring an alternative term such as "null" or "nonpositive" to emphasize that the finding of a lack of elevation of cancer risk is compatible with both the lack of any carcinogenic risk and with the qualitative presence of a risk of limited magnitude. Reflection on this issue makes clear that, even though one is evaluating the evidence on a qualitative question (Is the agent a human carcinogen?) based on qualitative attributes of study outcome (positive vs. negative), one cannot completely separate this issue from the quantitative question of the agent's potency. Studies meant to detect the "qualitative" property of carcinogenicity can in reality only do so according to limits set by the agent's potency and the statistical power of the study to detect effects of modest magnitude. This problem applies to animal studies as well as to human studies, but the lower power of epidemiological studies makes them bear the impact of the issue.

Returning to the case of an agent with "positive" animal results and "negative" epidemiological findings, then, one can distinguish two logical possibilities. First, there could, in truth, be no human hazard, the discrepancy being due to species differences (or dose level differences, or the route of administration differences) that make the agent a hazard to the animals but not to humans. Alternatively, there may indeed be a human hazard, but one of sufficiently modest potency that the epidemiological studies cannot detect, owing that to an insufficiency of power.

These two possibilities have profoundly different consequences for the assessment of human risks. In the absence of means to differentiate between them, the presumption is usually made that the more powerful animal tests detect a response that is shared with humans, which the less powerful human studies have simply failed to detect. It is this phenomenon that constitutes the issue of "ignoring epidemiology in risk assessment." Given the importance of this question, what evidence can be brought to bear to help distinguish between human studies that genuinely contradict and refute animal results and those that simply fail to detect the phenomenon seen in animal results?

The ambiguity of interpretation arises because of the *prima facie* case for potential human risk made by the existence of the animal responses. Thus, information casting doubt on the relevance of those responses to any potential human hazard, by undermining that *prima facie* case, tends to render the detectability question moot. The proposed revisions of EPA's Carcinogen Assessment Guidelines (EPA, 1994) call for much greater attention to the evaluation of the understanding of the mechanisms of tumorigenesis underlying animal results; if the physiological processes responsible for the tumors in animals can be shown to be qualitatively different in humans, such that the tumorigenic processes would not be expected to occur, then those animal tumors do not contribute to the weight of evidence for the agent's carcinogenicity in humans.

To the extent that this qualitative resolution cannot be obtained, the question must be approached quantitatively. That is, one must ask whether the observed results of the epidemiological studies *contradict* the animal-based projections of human risks. The concept is straightforward: if one can show that, were the risks implied from animal results to be true, the epidemiological studies would have shown detectable risks, then the lack of such detectable risks indicates that humans must in actuality be subject to much lower risks than the *prima facie* case from animals would indicate. In carrying out these calculations, however, a number of practical difficulties are encountered:

- Epidemiological studies often have poor quantitative characterization of exposure. Accordingly, it may be difficult to apply an animal-based potency (risk per unit of exposure) to calculate the hypothetical study results that would be obtained were the animal-based potency true.
- Unlike experimental animals in bioassays, the human subjects of epidemiological studies are usually followed for less than a full lifetime. The animal-based projection of full lifetime risk, then, must be corrected for that portion of the total lifetime risk that has yet to appear. There are ways to approximate such adjustments, but they invariably require additional assumptions about how late-in-life risks will be manifested.
- The definition of "risk" in human and animal studies is usually different in important ways. Although the same word is used, and the intended meaning is similar, the actual measures may not be compatible. For instance, human cancer risks are typically measured using mortality data (where the tumor is listed as cause of death), while incidences in animal studies include tumors (perhaps even benign tumors) discovered at terminal sacrifice among outwardly healthy animals. Human risks are defined vis-à-vis background risks of referent populations as played out in the gradually diminishing survivorship of life tables, while animal risks are defined vis-à-vis concurrent controls with terminal sacrifice at the end of a "conventional" lifetime.
- Animals are rigorously randomized among dose groups in bioassays, but the exposed groups in epidemiological studies may be subject to the "healthy worker effect," decreasing the apparent potency of agents.
- The anatomical sites at which tumors appear in animals may be different than the sites in humans. (The problem of "site concordance" in cancer risk assessment is perplexing; a further discussion is found below.) There is a question as to whether the most appropriate human-animal comparison should be on the basis of total risk, on the most sensitive site in each species, or on corresponding sites in animals and humans.
- There are questions about how properly to test for incompatibility of the human and animal results. That is, what outcomes constitute refutation of the animal-based potency projection by the results of the epidemiological studies?

This last point bears some further discussion. Because the limited power of the epidemiological study to detect an effect is what gave rise to the question, the "refutation" issue is sometimes asked in the same terms, i.e., does the human study have the power to detect a true risk of the magnitude predicted by the animal studies?

The power calculation, however, provides an answer to the wrong question. The statistical power issue arises in the *design* of studies and refers not at all to any actual study outcomes. The power question asks how large a *future* study there must be to be reasonably certain of detecting an effect of a given magnitude. If one were setting out to conduct a human study to refute a given animal-based risk projection, this approach would be appropriate. But once a study has been done, the issue is not its design but rather its results.

The appropriate question in the present case is: If the animal-based projections of human risk were true, what would be the likelihood of obtaining the *observed* results of the epidemiological study? If this likelihood is very small (i.e., if it is very unlikely that so few cancers were observed, were the agent's potency indeed as high as implied by the animal data) then the human data constitute a refutation of the hypothesis that humans are indeed at as high a risk as the animal data seem to imply.

Given the practical difficulties noted above, this calculation is not completely straightforward. The question of how to make such animal-human risk comparisons needs further work and development. Dr Sielken's paper in this volume explores some of these issues, but it reveals the difficulty of describing a well defined rejection region for low likelihood human outcomes. The literature contains an interesting discussion in a series of papers comparing cancer risks from inhaled methylene chloride as determined in mouse bioassays and in well conducted occupational cohort studies (EPA, 1987b; Tollefson et al., 1990, 1991; Hearne et al., 1987; Hearne, 1991; Stayner and Bailer, 1993).

As a final point, I would like to return to the question of site concordance. The fundamental tenet of toxicology — that toxic reactions in experimental animals constitutes evidence that humans may exhibit similar responses — rests on the high degree of anatomical, physiological, and biochemical homology across mammalian species. (If this ability to generalize across species, at least as a starting point, were not widely believed, toxicology would be an esoteric science indeed, consisting largely of the study of diseases of rats and mice caused by exposure to substances they would rarely encounter outside the laboratory). Of course, within this broad pattern of overall similarity there are myriad species differences, qualitative as well as quantitative, that can influence the outcome of chemical exposure. These differences can manifest themselves in various ways. In some cases a toxic reaction can be quite species-specific, hinging on some unique feature of the susceptible species' physiology.

In carcinogen risk assessment, this general phenomenon is encountered as the issue of "site concordance." It is rare for carcinogens to give completely concordant results — to produce tumors at exactly same sites and only those sites — in all tested species. Even agents that are "positive" in a variety of test animals often result in different arrays of tumor types from one species to the next.

For example, examining the Carcinogenic Potency Database for chemicals positive in at least one species, Gold et al. (1991) showed that only about one half of agents were positive at the same site in both rats and mice. (And these agents merely had one site in common; other responses may be discordant.) Yet three-fourths of agents positive for *some* site in one species were positive for *some* site in the other. Although all of the agents classified as known human carcinogens (based on epidemiological studies) have positive animal studies as well, the animal responses are not always for the same cancer type. Of the agents classified as human carcinogens by IARC that were represented in the Carcinogen Potency Database, Gold et al. (1991) found that only 4 of 13 were positive at the equivalent site in mice and 7 of 16 in rats.

Looking at the data quantitatively yields a similar phenomenon. For instance, Allen et al. (1988) found that animal potency data did rather well (at least on average) in predicting the potencies of carcinogens in humans that are observed epidemiologically, even though the tumor sites were often different. Restricting the animal projections to those based on the same tumor types as seen in humans did not improve the correlation appreciably.

The question, then, is how *specific* should the agreement in bioassay results be expected to be? There are many interesting implications (mostly beyond the scope of this paper) for hazard identification of carcinogens. To what degree should concordance strengthen (or discordance weaken) our evaluation of potential human hazard? How much should concordance with animal results strengthen otherwise inadequate human epidemiological results?

These questions require further thought and study. We project toxicological phenomena to humans based on the presumption of homology, and the weaker the evidence that such homology determines the outcome, the weaker the rationale for extrapolation. On the other hand, carcinogenicity at a somewhat more general level (i.e., without the expectation of strict site concordance) is seen to be more reliably projected across species than are any specific reactions. One must not overlook the difficulties of detecting effects of lower magnitude (as discussed above) and the likelihood that basically common toxic mechanisms manifest themselves somewhat differently in different species, owing to physiological differences that merely modify (rather than obviate) toxic processes.

To conclude, the explicit comparison of the results of animal experiments and epidemiological studies is fundamental to the process of risk assessment. Although the comparisons are often made qualitatively, in fact it is difficult to separate these considerations from the quantitative question of the detectability of moderate risks in studies of practicable size. Methods for comparing animal and human results, especially methods for quantitative comparisons of apparent potencies, need further development but hold great promise. The emerging interest in elucidation of underlying mechanisms of toxic action as a means of improving risk assessment will greatly aid in the understanding and correct interpretation of animal-human toxicological differences.

132

References

Allen BC, Crump KS and Shipp AM. Correlation between carcinogenic potency of chemicals in animals and humans. Risk Analysis 1988;8(4):531–544.

EPA. The Risk Assessment Guidelines of 1986. U.S. Environmental Protection Agency. Office of Health and Environmental Assessment, Washington DC, Document No EPA/600/8–87/045, 1987a.

EPA. Update to the Health Assessment Document and Addendum for Dichloromethane (Methylene Chloride): Pharmacokinetics, Mechanism of Action, and Epidemiology (Review Draft). U.S. Environmental Protection Agency. Office of Health and Environmental Assessment, Washington DC, Document number EPA/600/8–87/030A, 1987b.

EPA. Workshop Report on EPA Guidelines for Carcinogen Risk Assessment: Use of Human Evidence. U.S. Environmental Protection Agency, Washington DC, Document number EPA/625/3–90/017, 1989.

EPA. Respiratory Health Effects of Passive Smoking: Lung Cancer and Other Disorders. U.S. Environmental Protection Agency. Office of Research and Development, Washington DC, Document number EPA/600/6–90/006F, 1992.

EPA. Air Quality Criteria for Oxides of Nitrogen. U.S. Environmental Protection Agency. Office of Research and Development, Washington DC, Document number EPA/600/8–91/049cF, 1993.

EPA. Draft Revisions to the Guidelines for Carcinogen Risk Assessment (Review Draft). U.S. Environmental Protection Agency. Office of Research and Development, Washington DC, Document number EPA/600/BP–92/003, 1994.

Gold LS, Slone TH, Manley NB and Bernstein L. Target organs in chronic bioassays of 533 chemical carcinogens. Environmental Health Perspectives 1991;93:233–246.

Hearne FT. Response to Tollefson et al. Risk Analysis 1991;11(4):569–571.

Hearne FT, Grose F, Pifer JW, Friedlander BR and Raleigh RL. Methylene chloride mortality study: Dose-response characterization and animal model comparison. J Occup Med 1987;29:217–227.

NAS. Risk Assessment in the Federal Government: Managing the Process. Washington, DC: National Academy Press, 1983.

Stayner LT and Bailer AJ. Comparing toxicologic and epidemiologic studies: methylene chloride – a case study. Risk Analysis 1993;13(6):667–673.

Tollefson L, Brown RN, Lorentzen RJ and Springer JA. Response to Hearne. Risk Analysis 1991;11(4): 573–574.

Tollefson L, Lorentzen RJ, Brown RN and Springer JA. Comparison of the cancer risk of methylene chloride predicted from animal bioassay data with the epidemiologic evidence. Risk Analysis 1990;10(3):429–435.

©1995 Elsevier Science B.V. All rights reserved.
The Role of Epidemiology in Regulatory Risk Assessment
J.D. Graham, editor.

133

Use of available epidemiological data to validate rodent-based carcinogenicity models

Gay Goodman

Department of Pesticide Regulation, Toxicology Branch, Sacramento, California, USA

Key words: animal testing, assessment, carcinogens, epidemiology, health, human, risk, testing.

Introduction

Quantitative health risk assessment for chemical compounds is based on the results of toxicologic testing in experimental animals. For noncancer end points, the aim is to predict the maximum safe exposure level in humans based upon the highest dose level at which no adverse effects are observed in the animals under test. For agents which increase the site-specific incidence of tumors in rodents, the additional aim is to predict the carcinogenic potency (i.e., cancer risk per unit dose) in humans. Performance of quantitative risk assessment permits the design of risk/benefit analyses and allows a regulatory agency to make risk management decisions. Federal agencies and other regulatory bodies mandate that quantitative risk assessment be performed on industrial chemicals, pesticides, drugs, combustion products, waste-site components, and other classes of chemical compounds. With the obvious exception of drug testing, there are no requirements that human data be gathered, even if substantial human exposure has already occurred. When epidemiological studies pertinent to an exposure of interest already exist, they are utilized only sporadically in quantitative risk assessment.

Limitations on the use of animal data in human health risk assessment

An animal strain or species used in toxicologic testing may or may not be a suitable model for human health effects. Because of underlying differences in absorption, metabolism, and physiological disposition, the toxicity of a foreign substance is often qualitatively different in humans and the test species:

- A given toxic end point of interest may be produced only in the test species (or only in humans).

Address for correspondence: Gay Goodman, California EPA, Department of Pesticide Regulation, Medical Toxicology Branch, 1020 N Street, Room 342W, Sacramento, CA 95814-5624, USA. Tel.: +1-916-324-3512. Fax: +1-916-324-3506.

Quantitative differences in metabolism also are known to occur:

— The test species may be much more (or less) sensitive than humans with respect to a particular toxic end point.

In addition, qualitative or quantitative differences in response may arise from the fact that the conditions of exposure obtained in the rodent bioassay are not similar to human exposure scenarios. For example, there may be discrepant responses if the compound in question was given as a single daily dose in rodents and human exposures are intermittent or continuous throughout the exposure period. Similar problems may arise when extrapolating from essentially continuous exposure in rodents (e.g., via drinking water, feed, or inhalation) to intermittent or sporadic exposures in humans. Inherent or exposure-related interspecies differences in response could conceivably lead to significant over or underestimation of human risk.

A regulatory requirement for interspecies comparison of the pharmacokinetics of potentially toxic compounds would decrease uncertainty in the interspecies extrapolation of risk. For any given chemical agent, the conduct of comparative studies increases confidence in the use of a particular animal model or else indicates that the available animal models are not useful at all for a given end point. In the latter instance, epidemiologic results would be extremely valuable. When sufficient human data are lacking (as is usually the case), all concerned would benefit if regulators learned the habit of communicating their highest priority data needs to epidemiologists.

The need for epidemiologic data in cancer and noncancer risk assessment

Whereas noncancer risk assessment is primarily an exercise in interspecies extrapolation, cancer risk assessment relies on both interspecies and high- to low-dose extrapolation. Two tenets of regulatory toxicology are the basis for these divergent strategies:
1. Adverse noncancer effects are considered to occur only upon exceeding a threshold dose; and
2. Cancer generally is considered to be a nonthreshold phenomenon. Even if a chemical compound is suspected of being a threshold carcinogen (e.g., because it lacks genotoxic activity and the incidence of site-specific tumors in rodents is elevated only at the highest dose tested), only in rare cases will the biological data available be sufficient to demonstrate mechanism. Lacking such biological data, epidemiologic studies are the only means available to validate or invalidate the use of nonthreshold dose-response models for predicting carcinogenicity in humans.

For noncancer end points, the maximum safe human exposure level will be underestimated if the animal model is more sensitive than the human, but the error is generally expected to be within an order of magnitude overall. Let us assume that a compound is neurotoxic in rats at a subchronic dose level of 10 mg/kg/day but not at 1 mg/kg/day and, if tested, would produce an adverse effect (perhaps neurotoxicity) in the average human exposed subchronically at 100 mg/kg/day or above. With regulatory margin-of-safety (i.e., uncertainty) multipliers applied to the rodent data, the maximum allowable exposure level in humans might be set at 0.001 mg/kg/day. One of the usual margin-of-safety multipliers is meant to account for a possible 10-fold *underestimate* of the human effective dose by the animal model. Thus, when the animal model *overestimates* the human effective dose by 10-fold as in our example, there is an extra 100-fold margin of safety built into the regulatory level, above and beyond the factors accounting for other uncertainties. This could be construed by some as an unnecessary regulatory burden.

For cancer risk assessment, use of an inappropriate animal model can potentially incur larger errors than those associated with noncancer risk assessment. Carcinogenic potencies derived, for example, at rodent dose levels of 10–100 mg/kg/day are often used to regulate human exposures to carcinogens at levels of 0.001 mg/kg/day or less. But if a compound were potentially carcinogenic in humans only above a threshold dose which is three or more orders of magnitude above a given regulatory level, then perhaps that regulatory level is far too stringent. Here too, epidemiologic data can have a large impact. The rest of this chapter will focus exclusively on risk assessment for cancer end points.

Intraspecies and interspecies variability in the response to similarly high dose levels

Interspecies extrapolation of (quantitative) cancer risk has been shown to be reasonably predictive, on average, between mice and rats (Crouch and Wilson, 1979; Goodman and Wilson, 1991a). Correlation or consistency with rodent carcinogenic potencies has also been shown for the cancer incidence associated with exposures in epidemiologic studies; however, human exposure levels were almost all within one to two orders of magnitude of the doses tested in rodents (Goodman and Wilson, 1991b; Allen et al., 1988). It would be wrong to deduce that average tendencies based on a limited number of high-dose comparisons are an indication that interspecies and intraspecies variability are unimportant to the interspecies extrapolation of high-dose carcinogenic potencies to low-dose cancer risk. On the contrary, it is clear that interstrain, intergender, and interspecies differences are important enough to produce significantly less than 100% concordance for high-dose carcinogenicity even among such closely related species as rats and mice. Furthermore, the poorest concordance for carcinogenicity between rats and mice is found among compounds which produce tumors only at a single site in a single sex (Ashby and Tennant, 1988); these are mostly nonmutagenic compounds and are the likeliest candidates for threshold carcinogenesis.

Current developments in the genetics of human cancer susceptibility reveal that environmental induction of a wide variety of cancers is highly dependent on inherited mutations in genes coding for metabolizing enzymes or those which affect tumor initiation, promotion, or progression directly (Shields and Harris, 1991). As the techniques of molecular epidemiology come into more widespread use by investigators of human cancer susceptibility, risk assessors will be forced to consider interindividual differences in genetic susceptibility. This is particularly true with respect to regulating occupational and other high-dose exposures; recent work indicates that genetic susceptibility to environmental carcinogenesis sometimes exerts the most influence at the highest exposure levels. For example, among women who are nonsmokers or light smokers, those who are slow acetylators (i.e., whose variants of the P_{450} family of cytochromes are poor metabolizers of specific chemical agents) are not at increased risk for breast cancer compared to rapid or normal acetylators. However, among women who are the heaviest smokers, the slow acetylator phenotype appears to be a meaningful risk factor for breast cancer (Shields, 1991).

The problem of high- to low-dose extrapolation

For some compounds, the high- to low-dose extrapolation aspect of cancer risk assessment may be an even greater source of uncertainty than the interspecies aspect. Cancer risk assessment often entails extrapolation from high-dose rodent bioassay data to the much lower doses experienced in many human exposure scenarios (e.g., ingestion of trace contaminants in food or water). Most often, a linearized multistage model is fit to the rodent data and is used to extrapolate over more than a few orders of magnitude in dose. The primary justification for this approach comes from the results of several "super" bioassays (each entailing a much wider range of doses and animals per dose group than are usual in a rodent bioassay) on a handful of strong mutagens, including 2-acetylaminofluorene (Staffa and Mehlman, 1979; Carlborg, 1981) and several nitrosamines (Peto et al., 1984; Ito et al., 1984). Thus, for mutagens, high- to low-dose intraspecies extrapolation has been validated in rodents over the dose ranges examined in the super bioassays; however, there is no guarantee that carcinogenic potency will extend linearly or even smoothly down to zero dose from the lowest of the high doses tested in any rodent bioassay. For nonmutagens, high- to low-dose extrapolation has not been validated either in rodents or in humans.

Discovery of potential mechanisms of threshold carcinogenesis (such as induction of cell proliferation) has been one of the driving forces behind current efforts to reform the risk assessment process. For example, the ability to induce cell proliferation (and not in vitro mutagenicity) has been shown to correlate with rodent carcinogenicity for a pair of closely related mutagens (Cunningham et al., 1991). The observation that some mechanisms of threshold carcinogenesis are highly species-specific (e.g., bladder tumorigenesis in male rats (Cohen, 1991)) has heightened interest in finding ways to improve human cancer risk assessment through incorporation of epidemiologic data.

Practical means to utilize epidemiological data in combination with animal data in cancer risk assessment

The results of epidemiologic cohort studies can be used both to quantify the human cancer risk of long-term (chronic) exposures and to validate or invalidate rodent-based cancer risk assessment models as applied to those exposures. In the following paragraphs, a step-by-step guide to the process is outlined. The reader is referred also to Goodman and Wilson (1991b) for an illustration of how to utilize negative epidemiologic results to set upper limits on human carcinogenic potency.

Choose the best epidemiologic study (without weighting)

It is difficult to imagine a more subjective process than the assignment of weights to a group of studies. Weighting schemes are often quite arbitrary, containing within them a hidden bias (intentional or otherwise) toward higher or lower risk estimates. In the presence of extreme bias, the uncertainty in weight assignments could easily become larger than the uncertainty associated with reliance on single-model estimates of risk.

Each epidemiologic study should be evaluated separately on its own merits. The best epidemiology study is the one that is the most informative. This study may be chosen subjectively based on loosely objective criteria such as length of exposure, length of follow-up, extent of exposure characterization, consideration of confounding factors, and the power of the study to detect an effect. The rest of the epidemiologic data base need not be ignored: one should return to it later to determine consistency with the results of the "best" study. If consistency is lacking, further investigation into possible sources of the discrepancy (through careful comparison of design and data analysis strategies, for example) would be indicated.

Choose the rodent tumor site of greatest sensitivity (unless there is sufficient reason to exclude)

Choice of a single rodent carcinogenic potency on which to base an assessment of human risk is often less straightforward than choosing the best epidemiologic study. If two or more animal bioassays have followed good laboratory practice (GLP), administered a similar range of doses, and utilized the same number of animals per dose group, there may be no "best" study. This situation commonly occurs when the NTP has followed a similar protocol for both sexes of each of two rodent species. Regardless of the number of studies of similar quality, regulatory policy typically dictates that the risk assessment be based on the most sensitive site in any sex/species group. This approach would appear to make sense only when the rodent species/sex/-site and dosing regime in question comprise a good model for human cancer risk. Yet it is not possible to thoroughly gauge the appropriateness of a given animal model without knowledge of the test compound's pharmacokinetics and mechanisms of carcinogenicity in the test species and in humans. Thus, an organ-specific suscep-

138

tibility which is particular to an inbred strain (e.g., liver tumorigenesis in the B6C3F$_1$ mouse) could warrant exclusion of the tumor response in that organ. In the absence of complete mechanistic and pharmacokinetic information, most rodent potency options cannot be discounted. However, choices can be narrowed somewhat using available exposure information. For example, tumorigenicity at sites local to the point of contact of a single daily dose (such as esophageal, forestomach, or tracheal tumors following gavage administration) could reasonably be excluded if human exposures do not entail similarly concentrated, localized exposures.

Lack of knowledge concerning pharmacokinetics and mechanism, however lamentable, is never an acceptable reason for obscuring data selection under the cloak of a weighting scheme. To avoid bias and hidden agendas in the choice of a rodent tumor response on which to base the risk assessment, it is far better to summon all of one's toxicological expertise and chemical-specific knowledge, make a choice, and explain it fully. I would argue that when data appropriate to the choice of the most suitable animal model are lacking, one should carry on with the convention of choosing the most sensitive site identified among all eligible animal experiments (with eligibility decided as pharmacokinetic, mechanistic, and other knowledge permit). This approach offers the advantage of reproducibility; competent toxicologists may disagree or agree with the outcome but their reasoning is up front, facilitating acceptance or rejection by any reviewer. Furthermore, the outcome is conceptually simple and readily upgradeable as new pharmacokinetic/mechanistic data become available. On the other hand, the introduction of a complex, software-intensive weighting scheme is an added complication, requiring considerable statistical sophistication; meanwhile, the outcome is likely to be too subjective to be reproducible.

Weighting is touted as a means of taking all of the data into account. However, calculating a crudely weighted average over the results in different species, strains, sexes, and tissues is not the only possible means of accommodating the larger data base. An alternative is to use the body of results obtained in all studies as a guide for interpreting the relevance to human carcinogenicity of the selected, site-specific potency. Evaluating the weight of evidence is one (qualitative) aspect of the process. If consistency among the data base is not found, this may be viewed by the objective toxicologist as a signal to rethink the appropriateness of the chosen animal model. Furthermore, by highlighting a chemical compound's failure to produce a consistent response among the test species, toxicologists could serve to stimulate acquisition of the kind of basic, relatively inexpensive, comparative pharmacokinetic data that should have been gathered even before the rodent carcinogenicity bioassay was initiated.

Construct a matrix of human cancer risk predictions based on the selected animal model

There is generally no strong reason for believing that any given dose-response model or method of describing or normalizing dose is superior to any other for predicting human cancer risk from animal tumorigenicity data. Therefore it is instructive to ask whether any set of models or other assumptions concerning dose produces human cancer risk estimates which are more consistent than others with the epidemiologic findings.

An attempt to fit the dose response at the chosen (often most sensitive) site can be made using the linearized multistage model, which is the usual regulatory default. If this model is not a good fit to the data or if the time dependence of tumor appearance suggests that a Weibull, multistage-Weibull, or some other model would be more appropriate, these can be tried also. Included in the model calculations can be a range of choices for dose parameters, including administered daily dose vs. peak or steady-state blood levels (if known); normalization of dose on the basis of body weight to the power of one, two-thirds, or three-quarters; and time-weighted-average vs. cumulative dose. Whenever possible, the set of rodent dose metrics analyzed should include whichever human dose metrics are being considered in the evaluation of the epidemiologic data (discussed below). The results of analyses using all dose-response models providing a reasonably good data fit can be presented as a matrix of solutions corresponding to each set of parameter choices (see Sielken, Chapter 13, this volume).

Estimate the cancer potency in the selected epidemiologic study

Ideally, human exposure levels will have been measured or estimated by the authors of the selected study. If no exposure data were reported, the risk assessor should nevertheless attempt to calculate an approximate range of exposure levels using accessory information such as vapor pressure or regulatory air standards for industry (Goodman and Wilson, 1991b).

The relevant, site-specific, cancer incidence and 90% confidence interval (CI) or some other metric of uncertainty should be obtained from the epidemiologic study results. If the probability of cancer is a function of exposure dose, duration, or follow-up, then more than one useful measure of incidence may be obtained. Each measure of cancer incidence can then be fit to a truncated multistage dose-response model which is first-order (i.e., linear) in dose. For example:

$$P(d) = 1 - [1 - P(0)] \exp\left(-\frac{\beta d}{1 - P(0)}\right) \tag{1}$$

where d is the daily dose in mg/kg averaged over a 70-year lifetime (in units of mg/kg), $P(d)$ is the site-specific probability of cancer at the end of lifetime dosing at dose d, $P(0)$ is the analogous probability at zero dose (i.e., background incidence), and β is the carcinogenic potency (slope) (Crouch and Wilson, 1979). When $P(0) = 0$, this model reduces to:

$$P(d) = 1 - \exp(-\beta d). \tag{2}$$

If the site-specific background incidence is approximately 5% or less, then Equation 2 is a good approximation for Equation 1 (Goodman and Wilson, 1991b). For tumors which are more common than that, use of Equation 1 is indicated and therefore background incidence data must be obtained.

If the exposure duration was less-than-lifetime in the epidemiologic study selected then the results are not strictly comparable with the rodent bioassay results. Averaging dose over a lifetime is one means of attempting to compensate for shorter exposure durations; however, particularly for subchronic or intermittent exposures, other metrics may be more appropriate than the lifetime averaged dose. The risk assessor can perform additional analyses using, for example, cumulative dose, peak dose, or average exposure-period dose. Insertion of a time- and/or age-dependent correction to the relationship between the observed tumor incidence and dose may also increase the comparability of less-than-lifetime human exposure outcomes and rodent bioassay data (Goodman and Wilson, 1991b). The Armitage-Doll analysis of site-specific human cancer incidence revealed that the rate generally climbs with age raised to a power of between four and seven (Armitage and Doll, 1954). A time- and age-dependent correction based on the Armitage-Doll model can be made, choosing whether one wishes to err on the side of possible over- or underprediction of risk, with the highest risk predicted by the lowest power of age or time as a fraction of a lifetime. Based on Equation 2, the correction might take the form:

$$P(d) = 1 - \exp\left(-\frac{\beta d}{2}\left[\left(\frac{t}{70}\right) + \left(\frac{\tau}{70}\right)^4\right]\right) \tag{3}$$

where t is the exposure duration and τ is the age at the end of follow-up ($\tau \leq 70$), both in years, and d is the average, daily, exposure-period dose (in units of mg/kg). One should keep in mind that the shorter the exposure and the younger the subjects, the greater the uncertainty associated with extrapolation out to lifetime (or 70-year) exposure. Although it may be difficult to quantify this uncertainty, an attempt should be made to estimate its importance based on available data for the chemical compound under investigation or related compounds.

Equation 3 or a similar relationship can then be solved for the cancer potency (β) and a suitable CI. A model which is first-order in dose (such as those described by Equations 1–3) is sufficient when there is a single exposure level, an approximation of which may be the only exposure information available. In the unlikely event that multilevel exposure data are available and a biphasic (or multiphasic) dependence of cancer incidence on dose is observed, then the same model can be used to solve for the dose-dependent potency independently for each phase. It is unnecessary to use a model which includes higher order terms in dose because the cancer incidence will be essentially linearly dependent on dose in a narrow range around each dose level and perhaps beyond. Extrapolation to doses below or above those which occurred in the study is not the object of this exercise and thus is not a consideration in the choice of a dose-response model. Of course, one expects that linear extrapolation of human cancer risk over, say, one order of magnitude in human dose will introduce less error than a similar extrapolation over several orders of magnitude in animal dose.

A cancer potency and CI should be derived from the epidemiologic data irrespective of whether the attributable risk is positive, negative, or zero by standard statistical criteria. Statistical limitations of the study (e.g., less than lifetime exposure of less than 100,000 persons) may preclude the observation of significantly elevated risk, but an upper confidence bound may reveal consistency with the outcome of other epidemiologic studies nonetheless. If there is a lack of consistency among the epidemiologic data base, an attempt should be made to reconcile the differences, taking known confounders, exposure levels, characteristics of the study populations, and statistical issues into consideration, among other things. If the inconsistency cannot be resolved, the extent to which confidence in the selected study is eroded, if at all, must be addressed.

Reconcile the epidemiologic and animal results

The following question can now be asked: Is any subset of the matrix of derived rodent cancer potencies consistent with the human cancer potency/CI calculated from the epidemiologic study results? If so, then the analysis has provided evidence that, for the chemical compound under investigation, specific methods of extrapolating from rodent to human potencies are more appropriate than others. Joint analysis of rodent and human data similar to those described here will help define the conditions (e.g., of human exposure dose and duration) and the classes of compounds for which the rodent bioassay may be a useful predictor of human cancer risk. Further, they will give either a boost or a black eye to any subset of parameters or models used as the default by any given regulatory agency. In the complete absence of consistency between the rodent and human data sets, the risk assessor is left to pursue other lines of evidence which might either substantiate or cast doubt on the relevance of the human and/or rodent results. In particular, the analyst may now be in a good position to recommend what types of additional information (e.g., comparative pharmaco-kinetics, molecular epidemiology) would decrease the uncertainty surrounding cancer risk assessment for the compound of interest.

Utilizing the epidemiology of the future in cancer risk assessment

The epidemiologic studies referred to thus far in this chapter might be described as "premolecular." As such, the exposures are often poorly defined and the genetic variability of the study population is not addressed. By contrast, the epidemiology of the future will rely on precise molecular biomarkers of exposure and genetic susceptibility, resulting in far greater power to detect (or reject) the carcinogenicity of environmental exposures. Performance of one or more prospective epidemiologic studies will generally be necessary in order to validate the relationship between a

142

suspected exposure or susceptibility biomarker and cancer outcomes (Groopman and Kensler, 1993). Once validated, the biomarker can be used in less costly epidemiological designs, such as retrospective or case-control studies. A good example of the importance of molecular exposure biomarkers to the detection of an effect of chemical exposure on cancer outcome is the aflatoxin story. A study of hepatocellular carcinoma cases revealed no statistically significant relationship with aflatoxin exposure as determined by food-frequency interview; however, urinary markers of aflatoxin revealed a striking relationship. The same study demonstrated the importance of coexposures (hepatitis B virus, in this case) to chemical carcinogenesis in humans (Qian et al., 1994).

Molecular epidemiology not only offers an improved means to assess cancer risk in humans directly but also provides a laboratory in which to test mechanistic hypotheses concerning environmental carcinogenesis. Feedback between molecular epidemiologic evidence and experimental results in animals will facilitate development of a new generation of improved laboratory testing protocols for predicting the carcinogenic risks of chemical exposures in humans.

References

Allen BC, Crump KS and Shipp AM. Correlation between carcinogenic potency of chemicals in animals and humans. Risk Anal 1988;8:531–544.

Armitage P and Doll R. The age distribution of cancer and a multi-stage theory of carcinogenesis. Br J Cancer 1954;8:1–12.

Ashby J and Tennant RW. Chemical structure, *Salmonella* mutagenicity and extent of carcinogenicity as indicators of genotoxic carcinogenesis among 222 chemicals tested in rodents by the U.S. NCI/NTP. Mutation Res 1988;204:17–115.

Carlborg FW. 2-Acetylaminofluorene and the Weibull model. Fd Cosmet Toxicol 1981;19:367–371.

Cohen SM. Cell proliferation and bladder tumor promotion. In: Butterworth BE, Slaga TJ, Farland W and McClain M (eds), Chemically Induced Cell Proliferation: Implications for Risk Assessment. New York: Wiley-Liss, 1991;347–355.

Crouch E and Wilson R. Interspecies comparison of carcinogenic potency. J Toxicol Environ Health 1979;5:1095–1118.

Cunningham ML, Foley J, Maronpot RR and Matthews HB. Correlation of hepatocellular proliferation with hepatocarcinogenicity induced by the mutagenic noncarcinogen:carcinogen pair — 2,6- and 2,4-diaminotoluene. Toxicol Appl Pharmacol 1991;107:562–567.

Goodman G and Wilson R. Predicting the carcinogenicity of chemicals in humans from rodent bioassay data. Environ Health Perspect 1991a;94:195–218.

Goodman G and Wilson R. Quantitative prediction of human cancer risk from rodent carcinogenic potencies: A closer look at the epidemiological evidence for some chemicals not definitively carcinogenic in humans. Regul Toxicol Pharmacol 1991b;14:118–146.

Groopman JD and Kensler TW. Molecular biomarkers for human chemical carcinogen exposures. Chem Res Toxicol 1993;6:764–770.

Ito N, Shirai T, Fukushima S and Hirose M. Dose-response study of urinary bladder carcinogenesis in rats by N-butyl-N-(4-hydroxybutyl)nitrosamine. J Cancer Res Clin Oncol 1984;108:169–173.

Peto R, Gray R, Brantom P and Grasso P. Nitrosamine carcinogenesis in 5,120 rodents: chronic administration of 16 different concentrations of NDEA, NDMA, NPYR and NPIP in the water of 4,400 inbred rats with parallel studies on NDEA alone of the effect of age of starting (3, 6, or 20 weeks) and of species (rats, mice, hamsters). In: O'Neill IK et al. (eds), N-Nitroso Compounds:

Occurrence, Biological Effects and Relevance to Human Cancer, IARC Scientific Publications No. 57, Lyon: IARC, 1984.

Qian G–S, Ross RK, Yu MC, Yuan J-M, Gao Y-T, Henderson BE, Wogan GN and Groopman JD. A follow-up study of urinary markers of aflatoxin exposure and liver cancer risk in Shanghai, People's Republic of China. Cancer Epidemiol, Biomarkers and Prev 1994;3:3–10.

Shields PG and Harris CC. Molecular epidemiology and the genetics of environmental cancer. JAMA 1991;266:681–687.

Shields PG. Paper delivered at the 8th International Conference on Carcinogenesis and Risk Assessment (Genetics and Susceptibility: Impact on Risk Assessment), Barton Creek, Texas, November 30–December 3, 1994.

Staffa JA and Mehlman MA. Innovations in Cancer Risk Assessment (ED01 Study). Park Forest South, IL: Pathotox Publishers, 1979.

©1995 Elsevier Science B.V. All rights reserved.
The Role of Epidemiology in Regulatory Risk Assessment
J.D. Graham, editor.

The reliable use of epidemiology studies in regulatory risk assessments

Thorne G. Auchter

Director Institute for Regulatory Policy, Washington DC, USA

Key words: assessment, epidemiology, guidelines, parameters, regulation, risk.

Introduction

I would like to thank each participant for making the 1994 conference held at Lansdowne, Virginia entitled, The Proper Role of Epidemiology in Regulatory Risk Assessment, a success. The information that was produced by this conference will be valuable in laying the groundwork for suggested epidemiology guidelines. This paper will discuss the creation of guidelines for use of epidemiology studies in regulatory risk assessments.

The goal of this conference was to identify the issues that need to be addressed in order to reliably use epidemiology studies as a basis for regulatory decisions. During the ensuing discussions, it was pointed out that there exists a legal and moral responsibility between scientists and federal regulators which must be accepted when sharing factual information and drawing conclusions. Realizing that the responsibility rests not only with the scientific community that generated the study, but also with government agencies which use the study, this conference identified the following issues as critical for the use of epidemiology studies in regulatory risk assessments:
- Clarify the difference between regulatory risk assessments and other risk assessments.
- Define the role that scientific studies play in the development of regulation.
- Establish guidelines for the use of epidemiology in regulatory risk assessments.

The generation of this three pronged base has provided a solid foundation which will enable participants at the next conference to further develop reliable uses for epidemiology data in regulatory risk assessments.

The need for guidelines for epidemiology studies used in regulatory risk assessments

Regulatory risk assessments are considered separate from risk assessments performed

---

Address for correspondence: Thorne G. Auchter, Director, Institute for Regulatory Policy, 11 DuPont Circle, NW #700, Washington, DC 20036, USA. Tel.: +1-202-939-6976. Fax: +1-202-939-6969.

and used by other entities (i.e., scientists, members of the business community, environmental groups, educational institutions, nonprofit organizations and others). The most significant distinction, is that regulatory risk assessments need guidelines and parameters. This is due to the fact that a regulatory agency has a moral and legal responsibility to *all* individuals, under both their statutory authority and their statutory requirements, that could be compromised if scientific studies were misused or misinterpreted. When this fact is combined with the manner in which the studies are developed, there arises the potential for a negative impact on the public. For example, if farmers who grow the produce, sold in grocery stores, use pesticides which may leave a residue on the vegetables, and the federal government alerts the public to this fact, then the federal government announces that this pesticide residue may result in an increased risk of concern, but fails to explain how the reduced consumption of these foods is probably more detrimental than any potential risk from pesticide residue. This would be a breach of the duty that the federal government owes the American people.

Discussions stemming from the regulatory risk assessment distinction led to the conclusion that the scientific community needs a clearer understanding of how to effectively interact with federal regulators. Specifically, the circumstances under which scientific studies are being used must be clearly understood by the regulators, the scientists, and the public. Miscommunication between these groups will be minimized if a common language is employed, thus ensuring that everyone will understand how federal regulators are utilizing the scientific studies.

Once all interested parties realize that consistency among epidemiology studies is needed before they can be used reliably in regulatory risk assessments, focused guidelines for the regulatory agencies can be developed. Public knowledge of the role of epidemiology in regulatory risk assessments will enhance the use of epidemiology and will help the public keep the results of risk assessments in a proper perspective. Since there are two distinct phases for the use of epidemiology studies in risk assessments, there should be two correlating phases in the guidelines:

– Creation and execution of epidemiology studies used by regulatory agencies.
– Methodologies employed to analyze the resulting epidemiology data used by regulatory agencies.

The development of these guidelines will bridge the visible gaps between the scientific and regulatory communities, as well as between the regulatory community and the public interests it represents.

The creation and execution of epidemiology studies

The first phase is the creation and execution of the epidemiology surveys that are going to be used by regulatory agencies. In order for the data to be useful in regulatory risk assessments, it must be collected in a consistent manner. For example, prior to the initiation of the study, the parameters of the study, including the confidence interval to be used, should be defined and documented. Also, it is at this time that potential biases and confounders should be addressed by the researcher; this will allow for a more consistent approach to the issues.

Another area of concern is the publication of the study by the researcher. If the study is to be used for regulatory purposes, the published study should contain all data and conclusions gathered by the researchers. This would prevent selective use of the study at a later point in time. Additionally, the data published in the study should include the researcher's interpretation of the uncertainties inherent in the study. This could be used as a guide for those individuals and agencies who later interpret and use the study.

Recognizing that a possible biological mechanism, or biological plausibility, helps the study establish credibility, biological plausibility has become an important criteria in determining causation. For this reason, the statement of a biological mechanism needs to be based on established guidelines to ensure consistency among studies.

Exposure data are of utmost importance to regulatory risk assessments; the conclusions drawn by federal regulators for each study should be based on actual exposure data, alternatively, appropriate biomarkers could be used. The relative risk calculation should represent the type of exposure data used.

Although this is not a complete list of items that need to be addressed in phase one of the guidelines, it does provide insight to the types of concerns that need to be addressed before epidemiology studies can be effectively used by regulators.

The methodologies employed to analyze epidemiology data

The second phase of the guidelines should focus on the methodologies employed by federal regulatory agencies to analyze the data produced by the epidemiology studies. The reliability of epidemiology studies at low relative risks needs to be examined in detail due to the current debate regarding the appropriate levels at which epidemiology study results become suspect, and lose their reliability. This is an important issue that warrants serious attention because of the inaccuracies that could result from the misinterpretation of low relative risks.

Meta-analysis, a technique that combines the results from "similar" individual studies, raises several questions regarding the studies that can be used for this analysis and the accuracy of results produced via this technique. Confusion arises when conflicting definitions of the word "similar" are employed. Another consideration is the inaccuracy of the results when *dissimilar* studies are combined. Guidelines need to be established regarding this issue, as well as the appropriateness of using meta-analysis for regulatory risk assessment. Knowledge of the conditions for using a meta-analysis and when it will likely be used, would be beneficial to the researchers if they had that information prior to the design of their study. This will ensure consistent value of risk assessments used for regulatory purposes.

The P-trend test is used to describe the consistency of the observed outcome with a series of relative risk values. Some people claim that the P-trend test can be used as a surrogate for a dose-response curve. The accuracy of this claim needs to be examined, and if it is determined that the P-trend test can serve as a surrogate for the dose response curve, guidelines need to be established that will clearly enumerate the circumstances that will produce an accurate result.

It is evident from this discussion that in order for epidemiology studies to be used in a consistent manner by federal regulatory agencies so that all affected parties will be treated fairly, guidelines need to be adopted which will promote communication among the scientists, the federal regulators and the public. The communication will be in the form of reasonably consistent processes for the design of studies by the researchers, and the use of studies by the agencies.

©1995 Elsevier Science B.V. All rights reserved.
The Role of Epidemiology in Regulatory Risk Assessment
J.D. Graham, editor.

The proper role of epidemiology in regulatory risk assessment: reaction from a regulator's perspective

Thomas A. Burke

Johns Hopkins School of Hygiene and Public Health, Baltimore, Maryland, USA

Key words: assessment, dose-response, epidemiology, hazard, information, regulation, risk, toxicity.

The papers, presentations and discussions during this conference have made two things clear. Firstly, there is a critical need to refine the use of epidemiology in regulatory decision making. Secondly, epidemiologists need to establish a dialogue with regulators and regulatory risk assessors to develop approaches for improving the role of epidemiology. The development of guidelines for the proper use of epidemiology in regulatory risk assessment may be an important step in addressing these needs.

As an epidemiologist and former regulator, I have watched, in disappointment, during the past 15 years as the toxicology based risk assessment model has become the dominant decision tool in regulatory risk management. Even when human data have been available, animal models have often dominated federal and state efforts to regulate risk. The introductory paper by John Graham, through examination of the IRIS database, clearly illustrates the general failure of the regulatory process to incorporate epidemiological results into regulatory risk assessments.

Yet, in listening to the proceedings of these two days, it is also evident that historical approaches to epidemiological study design have not adequately addressed the needs of contemporary regulators. While the unique capabilities of epidemiological studies to identify human health risks were reaffirmed, so too were the methodological limitations of the field. The current environmental laws often require regulators to define "acceptable risks" or "no adverse effect levels". While epidemiology has been very useful in identifying hazards, few studies can provide the kind of dose-response information which has become so critical to the regulatory process. The challenge for the epidemiology community is to bridge the gap between historical study design approaches and contemporary information needs. The first step is understanding those needs.

Address for correspondence: Thomas A. Burke, Assistant Professor of Health Policy and Management, 551 Hampton House, Johns Hopkins School of Medicine, 720 Rutland Avenue, Baltimore, MD 21205, USA. Tel.: +1-410-955-1604. Fax: +1-410-614-2797.

Table 1. Examples of regulatory agency decisions.

No action — Accept risk
Listing — Identification of a hazard
Investigation — Decision to learn more
Communication — Inform public, workers, policy makers
Standard setting — Determination of acceptable risk
Ban — Determination of unacceptable risk
Emergency response — Short term risk prevention

The data needs depend upon the nature of the decision

Epidemiologists, by training, are expert critics. Indeed, the deliberations of this conference demonstrate just how aware epidemiologists are of the inherent uncertainty of their trade. The complexities of human beings, including unknown ranges of individual susceptibility and exposure, genetic diversity, competing disease risks, and unique lifestyle factors, introduce uncertainty into even the most well designed epidemiological investigations. Given these uncertainties, can epidemiology realistically contribute to the regulatory process? The answer is absolutely yes, particularly when the goal is risk prevention, not risk prediction.

The quality of data which are acceptable for risk management is widely variable. It often depends upon the nature of the decision and the availability of information on health risks. The following is a list of the range of decisions which health and regulatory agencies are called upon to make.

Clearly, all of these actions do not require the same degree of data quality. In fact, few of the routine decisions of such agencies actually require specific quantitative point estimates of population health risks. In the large majority of instances, epidemiology can, and indeed does, serve a valuable role in guiding the actions of risk managers.

The lack of available human data for many hazards are perhaps a bigger problem than the challenge of proper use of epidemiologic results. In practice, regulators often are forced to make decisions with little or no data on potential adverse health effects in humans. Speaking from personal experience, I recall instances involving suspected product tampering, food contamination, and environmental emergency response where quick decisions were necessary to safeguard the public, yet there was virtually no epidemiological information to guide decisions. In these instances, because of the potential for widespread acute health impacts, drastic short-term protective actions are often taken with little or no controversy.

In contrast, there are other instances where public concern or high costs of control or remediation drive the demand for seemingly endless research and evaluation to develop detailed quantitative estimates of potential population health impacts before decisions are made. The ongoing controversy surrounding dioxin in the environment is an example of the latter case. In this case, over a billion dollars have been spent to evaluate the health risks of dioxin exposure. However, the research, which includes a number of epidemiological studies, has failed to result in a regulatory strategy to effectively address remediation of the environment or prevention of human exposure.

As the dioxin case demonstrates, health risk is not the only factor which drives the regulatory process. There are important social, political, and economic considerations which also drive regulatory decisions. Table 2 points out some of these factors. The arrows represent the variable nature of these drivers which may change as scientific information becomes available or as public concern shifts.

As the table points out, different factors will drive each decision. In addition, the strategies are often different at the federal, state, and local levels. Realistically, even a refined approach to epidemiology will not drive the regulatory process. Rather, the role of epidemiology is to inform the participants and guide the development of risk management strategies.

The role of epidemiology in risk characterization

The proceedings of the conference indicate that perhaps the most valuable contribution of epidemiology in regulatory risk assessment is in the risk characterization step of the process. While most human studies may currently lack the capability to determine specific dose response relationships, they offer important qualitative validation to the risk assessment. In addition, as Gene Matanoski's paper describes, epidemiology can address a much broader range of human health effects than current animal models, and offers insight into the potential public health impacts at the actual levels to which the human population is exposed.

The work of Robert Sielken offers approaches for combining human and animal studies in the characterization of risks. Such an approach could be used to characterize the plausibility of risks and allows direct inclusion of both qualitative and quantitative studies. By suggesting ways to use epidemiology to weight animal based predictions, Sielken provides a novel approach which may help to address the current

Table 2. Examples of factors which drive regulatory decisions.

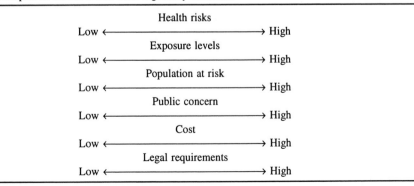

152

weaknesses in animal-based predictions of human risk and improve interspecies extrapolation.

On a more cautionary note, Suresh Moolgavkar points out the unenviable task of the regulatory risk assessor warning that we may never be able to predict the dose of an agent which increases lifetime risk by 1 in a million. However, he explains that the goals of the regulator do not necessarily coincide with those of the epidemiologist and notes that the criteria for use of epidemiologic data should be flexible depending upon the nature of the decision to be made.

At the current time, there is growing support for expansion of the characterization of risk in regulatory risk assessments. Activities range from agency specific guidelines on presenting risk estimates to proposed legislation to promote a more robust presentation of potential population risks. In addition, the National Academy of Sciences has convened a Committee on Risk Characterization, which is developing a report on improving current risk characterization methods in regulatory risk assessments. Expanded application of epidemiology in risk assessment has the potential to contribute to the refinement of current risk characterization practices and improve the public health basis for risk decisions.

Consensus on the role of risk assessment?

To say that this conference did not reach consensus on specific approaches to the use of epidemiology in regulatory risk assessment would be an understatement. In fact, the sessions were filled with vigorous discussion, frequent disagreement, and more than a little criticism of the current state of epidemiology and its applications for risk management. However, amidst the arguments, certain themes did emerge which I have attempted to summarize in the following list:
— Epidemiology is essential to the risk assessment process if we are to strengthen the public health basis for regulatory decisions.
— Current regulatory risk assessment practices lack an appropriate framework for the consideration of available epidemiological data.
— In general, there is a paucity of epidemiological data on many of the hazards which confront regulatory agencies at the federal, state, and local levels.
— The historical design of epidemiologic investigations have been aimed at identifying hazards and often do not provide adequate information on exposure or dose to derive quantitative estimates of population risks.
— Although they share a common goal of understanding and reducing human health risks, risk assessors and epidemiologists have not worked together to address the needs of regulators.
— Epidemiologists could increase the application of human data in risk assessment through improved consideration of the data needs of risk assessors and regulators.
— Establishment of guidelines for the use of epidemiology in risk assessment, developed to allow flexibility in their application, may offer an opportunity to advance the discipline and improve the consideration of human data in the

evaluation of risks.
- The role of epidemiology data on human health risks will become increasingly important as the nation moves toward wider use of the risk assessment process to guide national priorities.

Conclusions

Epidemiology is the core science of public health. However, in the past 15 years the fundamental role of epidemiology has been supplanted by an increasing dependence upon animal-based models to assess many environmental health risks, particularly cancer risks. At the present time there is an increasing need to develop improved approaches to evaluating and regulating noncancer health risks. This challenge may represent an unprecedented opportunity for epidemiologists to participate in reshaping regulatory risk assessment. Perhaps the time has come for the epidemiology community to wake up and smell the coffee, and recognize the critical importance of the proper application of human studies to the nation's regulatory efforts.

Never before has there been a greater dependence on risk assessment to guide regulatory decisions, yet at the same time there is growing dissatisfaction with the limitations and uncertainties of current approaches. Fundamental questions concerning the relevance of animal data to the human experience continue to undermine the credibility of many regulatory decisions. Presently, institutions ranging from the National Academy of Sciences to the U.S. Congress are grappling with approaches to improve the characterization and management of risks. Refining the role of epidemiology should be a key component of these efforts.

Among the participants in this conference there was understandable apprehension about the development of guidelines for the application of epidemiology in risk assessment. Will they become a rigid report card for epidemiology studies? Will they discourage flexibility in the design of investigations? Will they lead to further guidelines on the conduct of epidemiology? These are important concerns which must be addressed before any guidelines could be adopted.

On the other hand, guidelines or not, epidemiology is currently playing an increasing role in contemporary regulatory issues. From water chlorination to breast implants; electromagnetic fields to environmental tobacco smoke; results of epidemiologic studies are being used by regulators to guide decisions. Shouldn't epidemiologists participate in determining how their data are applied?

The development of guidelines may prove to be a valuable catalyst for beginning a long overdue dialogue between epidemiologists and regulatory risk assessors. The effective use of epidemiology in risk assessment will require a rethinking of traditional approaches to better address contemporary regulatory needs. It may also require the development of new approaches to the training of both risk assessors and epidemiologists. The challenge is clear. Risk assessment is here to stay and its applications for priority setting and regulation will continue to grow.

The risk assessment train is leaving the station, the Congressional, number 104.

Perhaps the development of guidelines will be the ticket for the epidemiology community to get on board and play a leadership role in reshaping the national approach to evaluating and preventing public health risks.

Index of authors

Keyword index